ETERNAL HEALTH

ETERNAL HEALTH

MICHAEL ELSTEIN M.D.

NACSON & SONS PTY LTD

Published by Nacson & Sons Pty. Ltd.
P.O. Box 515, Brighton-Le-Sands NSW 2216
Telephone: +61 (02) 9281 6178   Facsimile: +61 (02) 9281 2075

Copyright©2000 Nacson & Sons Pty Ltd

Design by Eli Nacson
Illustrations by Andrew Davies
Edited by Claudia Blaxell
Front Cover Photography by Wendy McDougall
Printed and bound in Australia by McPherson's Printing Group

ISBN: 0-947266-44-5

TO MY MOTHER JACQUELINE
WHOSE ENORMOUS LOVE
FILLS THE PAGES OF THIS BOOK

Acknowledgments

I would like to thank Tim who continues to inspire me, Sharon who is always there for me, Arthur and Claudia for all the hard work they have put into this book as well as Leon and Eli. All those who have impacted positively on my life, you the reader whose commitment to health and wellbeing gives me great hope for the future of this wonderful planet and Bennie whose love illuminates every day of my life.

Contents

Foreword

WE ARE WITNESSING A RENAISSANCE IN THINKING ABOUT HEALTH and disease, and a revolution in health care is underway.

Doctors are changing the way they think about health and illness, but at the same time they are struggling against that change. Every day new information comes to light that upsets the old order, but the new order is not yet in charge. Powerful interests are at stake and billions of dollars are there to be made or lost.

Entire industries, including the pharmaceutical industry, the cancer industry and the cardiovascular surgery industry, are reeling under the shockwaves of medical advances. As scientific research continues to provide exciting new information, enlightened medicos everywhere are coming to the conclusion that perhaps their medical school education was based on limited paradigms. It is a painful realisation for doctors; one that is still resisted by many.

The renaissance medicos, who are still a minority but quickly increasing in number, are constantly under attack by the medical establishment, the government bodies that are keen to protect the system and the industries that pay the bills. But there is no stopping the millennium medicine movement.

The fastest growing areas of medicine beyond the year 2000 will clearly be those that have a common skein with ancient systems of healing, and which also utilise the technological advances of modern medical research and diagnostic techniques. Popular medicine in the new millennium will approach sickness as an issue of balance and relationship: the result of disharmony between the sick person and their lifestyle, environment, belief systems and genetic inheritance, rather than the product of specific diseases.

The new medicine views optimal health as much more than the absence of sickness. Health is seen as a state of wellbeing in which the individual's body, mind, emotions and spirit are in harmony with and guided by an awareness of society, nature and the universe. The trend in this exciting new field of 'integrative medicine' is to embrace the concept that genetic inheritance is merely the hard drive upon which we build our unique life experiences. Research now indicates that there is significant variation in how people respond to diet, lifestyle and even their daily thoughts. There is also overwhelming evidence to show that our body's functioning performance can be greatly enhanced by nutritional and holistic therapy support.

Dr Michael Elstein is one of those renaissance doctors that I would call a health specialist rather than a disease specialist. He focuses on health and healing and is concerned with improving the total wellbeing of his patients, rather than just treating their symptomatic flare ups. In particular, Dr Elstein is fascinated by the dynamic, cutting-edge research in the field of anti-ageing medicine that incorporates the use of nutrients to modulate the expression of our genes. Science is rapidly piecing together a fundamental understanding of the mechanisms of ageing. We now know that biological ageing and the diseases associated with growing old can be prevented through nutrition.

In Eternal Health, Dr Elstein provides a comprehensive layman's guide to this exciting area of medicine; an area that should interest us all. After all, doesn't everybody want to stay in good physical, mental and emotional shape for their entire journey?

Among numerous case histories I could mention here, I have watched a 40-year-old friend of mine regain the vitality and enthusiasm of his youth with Dr Elstein's help. My friend's tendency toward depression, negativity, impotency and lack of appetite were overcome in a dramatic fashion after he embraced a simple anti-ageing protocol aimed at improving his general health and supporting the hormone levels that had dropped as a result of biological ageing. Today, my friend is a picture of health and has a new lease on life.

I thoroughly enjoyed Eternal Health and I'm sure you will too. I can offer no greater tribute to Dr Elstein than to say he is a doctor with an open heart and an open mind who is willing to listen to his patients and friends. He is committed to helping people achieve and maintain a high level of wellbeing, find purpose in their lives and make a positive difference in the world.

ARTHUR STANLEY
Journalist, researcher and author of
Bursting the Allergy Bubble and *Mind Your Own Health*

CHAPTER 1

The Anti-Ageing Revolution

The Anti-Ageing Revolution

*W*ELCOME TO 21ST CENTURY MEDICINE. YOU ARE ABOUT TO embrace one of the most monumental changes that modern medicine has ever witnessed. For the very first time, physicians are focusing their attention on health and wellbeing rather than disease and infirmity. Preserving vitality has become the number one priority for a brave group of inspired doctors and scientists who are daring to thumb their noses at the way conventional medicine views reality. This has arisen from one of the most challenging aspects of everybody's life—growing old.

I don't know about you, but one of the things that terrifies me the most about ageing is losing my energy and vitality. I want to remain as well and exuberant as I can, and look and feel good for as long as possible. If you share this desire, and I believe that you secretly do, then you are about to discover information that will dramatically alter your ideas about ageing.

You see, until now, modern medicine has not concerned itself much with health. Consider what would happen if you approached your average physician with inquiries as to how you could achieve optimal health. If you told them you wished to reverse the ageing process, you would be received with a blank stare, as if you were asking for the impossible. However, if you broached the subject of one of the many textbook diseases, you would see their face light up.

The majority of doctors know about illness and they know about the drugs used to treat illness, but ask them about wellness and they can't help you. This is why the science of anti-ageing medicine was developed. Around the world, enlightened medicos are banding together to provide you with amazing insights as to how you can remain in robust health for as long as you desire. The wonderful thing about this revolution is that we are all in it together. For once we are all in the same boat, sharing the same fears, hopes and desires. Anti-ageing medicine does not separate the patient and the doctor. All of us want to maintain our health, none of us want to get sick, so when we talk to you we are also addressing ourselves.

How many of you are noticing that your memory is not what it used to be? How often do you come down with the flu and take a devilishly long time to shake it? Have you noticed that you are putting on weight with inexplicable ease, but when it comes to shedding those unwanted kilos, it's an impossible task? Is your hair line receding and your libido diminishing? Do you have less energy than you used to? These are the signs of ageing. What you are probably not aware of is that these events can be altered. You do not have to view ageing as a relentless slide into decrepitude and senility. You can halt and even reverse these changes if you take the appropriate action.

Anti-ageing medicine is all about providing you with the knowledge and wisdom that will allow you to enjoy a life of vitality and vigour well into old age. If you follow the recommendations in this book, you will become a participant in a worldwide revolution in health care. You will be one of the standard bearers of a reformation that promises to alter the way we view our health and wellbeing forever. All the factors associated with ageing such as loss of memory, independence, strength and agility are now considered imminently preventable. You can anticipate endless years of sexual vitality, mental clarity and boundless energy if you take the necessary steps. This kind of lifestyle is freely available. The crucial step that you have to take is to commit yourself to an anti-ageing program. I believe that if you want to optimise your health and experience all the benefits of longevity, then the only way forward is through such an undertaking.

Take a look at the statistics and you will realise how vital such a program is. At the moment, the chances of getting cancer are one in three. By the year 2000 this number will have increased to one in two. Intriguingly, when we take a look at cardiovascular health, the picture is very similar. For a 40-year-old, the risk of developing heart disease sometime in life is one in two for men and one in three for women. For a 45-year-old the likelihood of sustaining a stroke before the age of 85 is one in four for men and one in five for women. These statistics are telling us in no uncertain terms that precious few will negotiate the ageing process without suffering a severely crippling disease. These facts become even more alarming when we consider the demographic changes that are taking place in Western society.

The 65-and-over age group is the fastest growing segment of the population. These are also the people that are going to manifest the above mentioned diseases of ageing. This being the case, we simply won't have the funds to deal with such a problem. If the prevailing trends persist into the new millennium, and there is every likelihood that they will get worse, then we will witness an unprecedented crisis in health care delivery. Unless we change the health care model we will bankrupt the Medicare system and have an ageing population that will not be adequately looked after.

The exciting news is that this does not have to happen. Anti-ageing medicine can deliver us from this nightmare into a land of prolonged health and wellbeing well into old age. If ageing is a time when degenerative diseases are rife, then ageing itself can be viewed as a disease. What a fascinating thought—*ageing as a preventable and treatable disease*. By substituting the infirmity and lingering diseases of ageing with health and vitality, a catastrophe can be averted. Billions of dollars can be saved while healthy productive lives can be generated.

People often ask me when they should commence an anti-ageing program. I always reply that the time to start is now. If you want optimal health well into old age, you need to start off with a good foundation. Once you are on the right track from a very early stage, you will be able to steer yourself along the path to longevity, free of the diseases of ageing. If you want to live a longer, healthier life you need to be proactive. The truth is that you don't suddenly develop Alzheimer's disease, cancer or heart disease. These can take up to 20 years to fester in your body. You probably won't even be aware that these diseases are establishing themselves until it is too late. This is why you need to pay attention to the early indications of premature ageing. As you will discover, increasing fatigue, poor resistance to infections and a lack of energy are the early warning signs that your body is undergoing an untimely decline. Ignore these at your peril.

Remarkably, we don't know exactly what it is that causes ageing. Why is it that the cells of our bodies lose their recuperative and regenerative powers? What is it that robs us of our vitality and our ability to carry on forever? We may not have the answers to these mysteries yet, but there are certain indisputable processes that surround the circumstances of ageing. Firstly there is the accumulation of free-radicals, and secondly there is the well recognised decline in vital anti-ageing hormones, both of which are thought to have a major impact on ageing. Let's take a look at each of these factors in turn.

Free-Radicals And Ageing

The single biggest threat that we have to counter as we grow older is that of the dreaded free-radicals. There is a growing consensus that free-radicals are the initiators of just about every disease known to man, and ageing is no exception. One of the pioneers of anti-ageing medicine, the renowned Dr Denham Harman, claims that free-radical reactions are the primary cause of ageing. The neurodegenerative diseases such as Alzheimer's and Parkinson's disease, as well as cancer and heart disease, can be viewed as overwhelming free-radical catastrophes with which the body's defences are unable to cope. What exactly are these free-radical events and what can we do to defend ourselves against such a foreboding enemy?

Free-radicals are a by-product of the body's normal metabolic processes. Oxygen, together with carbohydrates, proteins and fats, provides the essential fuel that our cells use to generate energy. When oxygen is utilised in this fashion, the oxygen molecule loses an electron and this is when it becomes a free-radical. A free-radical is simply a molecule that has lost an electron in its outer orbit, whereas a normal oxygen molecule has electrons that travel in pairs. This creates a state of instability that free-radicals find intolerable. They attempt to restore balance by regaining the electron they miss from another molecule. In so doing, that molecule loses an electron and a chain reaction is set up, which results in the accumulation of hordes of free-radicals with massive destructive capabilities. One of the great paradoxes of life is our inability to survive without oxygen, yet oxygen has the potential to destroy us. It is the exposure to oxygen that makes the apple go brown, causes iron to rust and turns butter rancid. These very same processes are taking place in our cells on a daily basis, and this is what makes us increasingly susceptible to ageing.

The venue for the production of cellular energy is the mitochondrion. Every cell in the body contains an assembly of mitochondria that busily go about their daily functions, generating energy. All this frenetic activity, which depends on the utilisation of oxygen, leads to the build-up of an excessive amount of free-radicals that are hell bent on destroying the very tissue that created them. *Mitochondria are exceptionally vulnerable to the devastatingly destructive effects of free-radicals*. They have no repair systems, no protective coating and they are 2,000 times more susceptible to free-radical damage than the other components of your cells.

The number of mitochondria in your cells decreases with age. If you have a big night out and consume lots of rich food and alcohol and are exposed to cigarette smoke, you will also destroy a number of healthy mitochondria. What then happens is that you have a number of faulty mitochondria reproducing themselves, and the result is a woefully inadequate energy source for your cells. Imagine trying to light up your house with a number of tiny 1.5 volt batteries. It isn't possible. Once energy is not produced efficiently, cellular processes go into decline and age-related diseases are able to establish themselves. It is therefore reasonable to postulate that ageing and all the diseases that go with it, result from the progressive damage that mito-chondria sustain at the hands of free-radicals. As the body ages, there is an increase in the formation of free-radicals and a decline in available defences. With so much oxygen being consumed it is not surprising that free-radicals proliferate. What is needed is a means to withstand this pernicious onslaught.

Free-radicals are caused by the normal processes of the body, but they also increase with exercise or exposure to toxic chemicals, car exhaust fumes, pesticides, herbicides, cigarette smoke and all the other pollutants to which we are constantly subjected. This is where antioxidants come to the rescue. What antioxidants do is donate electrons in order to neutralise the effects of free-radicals. If degenerative diseases result from an imbalance between free-radicals and antioxidant defences, having a good supply of antioxidants will prevent the diseases of ageing from establishing themselves.

Antioxidants perform best when they operate synergistically. For example, when vitamin E neutralises a free-radical it loses an electron, and in doing so it becomes a free-radical itself. Vitamin C then steps in and rescues vitamin E by donating an electron, which allows vitamin E to continue its antioxidant activity. Vitamin C then becomes a free-radical and is dependent on another antioxidant for its regeneration. This operation is very similar to the way in which a team of basketball players interchange during a match, with players returning to the fray when they are rejuvenated. This is why you should take antioxidants that complement each other as each is dependent on the other for its survival and continued activity.

When it comes to antioxidants, the most crucial are those that protect the mitochondria. Coenzyme Q10, alpha lipoic acid, acetyl-l-carnitine, vitamin E and vitamin C are the most vital antioxidants as far as mitochondrial support is concerned. Together they form a veritable fortress against the ravaging onslaught of the free-radical hordes. If you can maintain the optimum health of your mitochondria, you will provide your cells with sufficient energy to continue their daily functions. This is one of the key ways to preserve health and vitality. These powerful antioxidants are mentioned repeatedly throughout this book, and you will discover how vital they are for your brain, heart and all the other organ systems of your body.

The Hormones

On a par with antioxidants, preserving youthful levels of certain key hormones is an essential part of any anti-ageing program. These substances determine whether we remain vibrant, happy and healthy, and whether we enjoy longevity.

Hormones are chemical messengers that are secreted by the endocrine glands, which control bodily processes. They tell our cells what to do and how to behave in a way that is similar to a coach instructing the members of a team. Hormones work in unison, and, together with the nervous system, orchestrate the function of more than 50 billion cells in our bodies.

The endocrine glands (hormone producers) such as the pancreas, thyroid, adrenals and pituitary, are relatively small in size yet their effects on our bodily functions are considerable. Digestion, sexuality and the workings of our heart, liver and kidneys are controlled by the endocrine glands. Whether we become fat or thin, tall or short, is regulated by our hormone levels. If our hormones are operating in harmony with each other, then all is well with our bodies and we are fit and healthy. As we grow older the performance of our endocrine glands tends to diminish and the characteristic signs of ageing such as weight gain, flabby muscles, wrinkled skin and fatigue begin to manifest. However, it is important to realise that these changes are not inevitable. There are a number of factors that are important for hormonal wellbeing. How effectively you nurture your endocrine glands will impact on how well they serve you as you age. Let's look at how the endocrine system works in more detail.

Like the conductor and the first violinist of an orchestra, the hypothalamus and the pituitary exert similar control over your hormonal system. These are two master glands located in your brain. The hypothalamus controls pituitary secretions as well as hunger, sex drive, thirst and body temperature. The pituitary controls bone growth and regulates the activity of the thyroid gland, adrenals, gonads and the rest of the reproductive organs. Figure1. illustrates where these endocrine glands are located in your body and includes the other components of your endocrine system. The hypothalamus and

The hormonal conductor leading the endocrine orchestra

pituitary are affected by your thoughts and feelings via chemical messengers called neurotransmitters. These are relayed by your nervous system so that your mental and emotional states profoundly influence the nature of your hormonal secretions. This is why you feel tired and your sex drive diminishes when you are mentally stressed. Likewise, if you think you are old, then your performance will be consistent with your expectations.

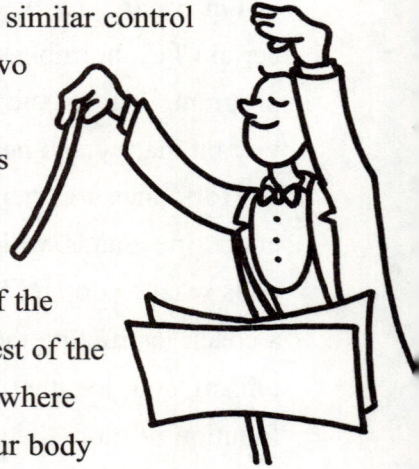

Maintaining optimal neurotransmitter balance has a significant effect on the workings of the hypothalamus. In Chapter 5 you will learn how these neurotransmitters can affect the development of neurodegenerative diseases.

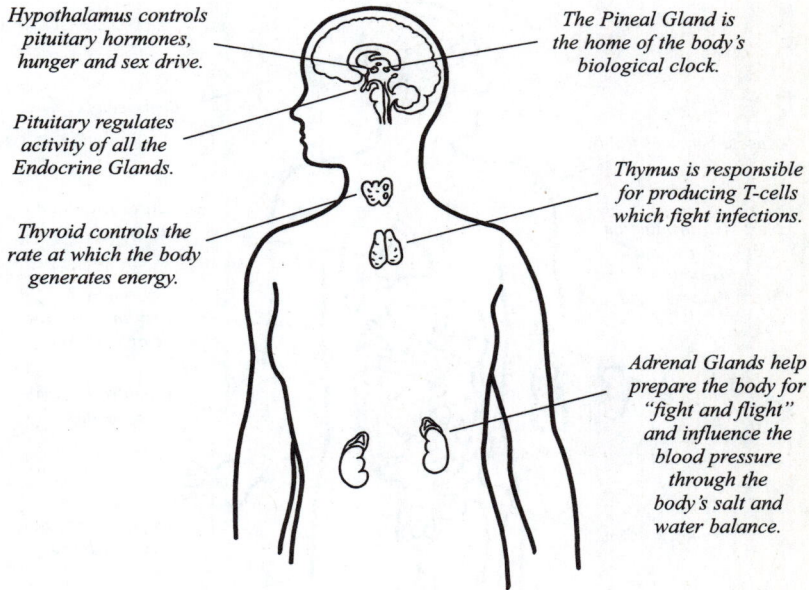

Hypothalamus controls pituitary hormones, hunger and sex drive.

Pituitary regulates activity of all the Endocrine Glands.

Thyroid controls the rate at which the body generates energy.

The Pineal Gland is the home of the body's biological clock.

Thymus is responsible for producing T-cells which fight infections.

Adrenal Glands help prepare the body for "fight and flight" and influence the blood pressure through the body's salt and water balance.

Figure 1.

Your hypothalamus influences the hormones that your pituitary secretes by means of releasing hormones. Once the pituitary receives a hormonal command from the hypothalamus, it secretes hormones that initiate various actions in the endocrine glands of your body.

The hypothalamus secretes gonadotropin-releasing hormone, which stimulates the release of follicle-stimulating hormone (FSH) and luteinising hormone (LH) from the pituitary. In women, FSH and LH control the menstrual cycle via the hormones oestrogen and progesterone. In men, FSH and LH promote the production of sperm and testosterone respectively. Thyroid hormone, growth hormone, the adrenal hormones and the rest of your endocrine system are all regulated in a similar fashion.

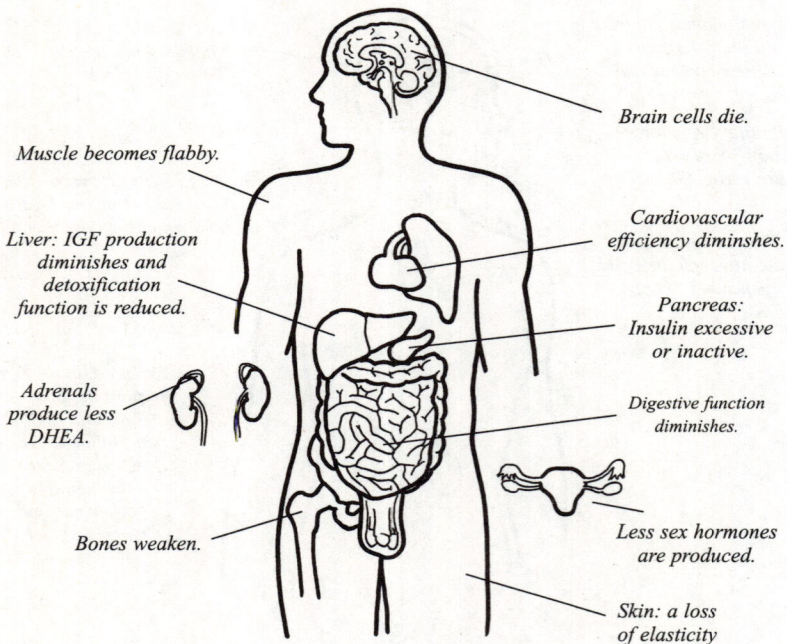

Brain cells die.

Muscle becomes flabby.

Cardiovascular efficiency diminshes.

Liver: IGF production diminishes and detoxification function is reduced.

Pancreas: Insulin excessive or inactive.

Adrenals produce less DHEA.

Digestive function diminishes.

Bones weaken.

Less sex hormones are produced.

Skin: a loss of elasticity

Figure 2. *What happens when we age?*

Figure 2 illustrates the decline in bodily function that occurs with ageing, and you can see that the contraction in organ activity parallels the weakening of the endocrine system. Most of the major changes that occur are due to a deterioration in hormonal activity. Oestrogen, DHEA, testosterone, growth hormone and thyroid hormone undergo age-related decline, and it is these hormones along with melatonin and testosterone that are targeted in the forthcoming chapters. Although we don't fully comprehend the reasons for this hormonal decline, what we do know is how to restore these hormones to their youthful levels, which is the essence of any anti-ageing program.

For the anti-ageing hormones to function optimally, they need to be sufficiently stimulated by the releasing hormones that emanate from your two master controlling glands—the hypothalamus and the pituitary. Whether these releasing hormones are received in the proper fashion by the receptor sites on the walls of your cells, depends on the friendliness of the environment. If it is too acidic the receptiveness of your cells will change and chemical messengers will be received less favourably. An alkaline environment is far more conducive to the activity of your messenger hormones. Maintaining a pH (which refers to the degree of acidity or alkalinity of your blood and cellular environment) whereby metabolic function can proceed efficiently, is an essential part of your anti-ageing strategy. A Biological Terrain Assessment is one of the new technologies for evaluating pH levels, and you will learn how you can incorporate this test in your anti-ageing program.

Endocrine glands that are exhausted by constant stress will eventually succumb and your hormone levels will start to decline. Therefore it is important to provide the building blocks for your cells to manufacture the hormones that your body needs. Hormones are made from proteins and fats such as fish, tofu, eggs, nuts, seeds and avocado. A healthy digestive system will present these nutrients to your cells in adequate amounts, and a healthy liver will process your hormones so that your body can eliminate them when they are no longer needed.

When you consider that your hormones perform synergistically like a finely-tuned symphony orchestra, you will realise that you have to start looking after your endocrine system from a very early age, and noticing the warning signs of hormonal imbalances. Fatigue, reduced libido and a lack of vitality should start the alarm bells ringing. This is an indication that urgent action is needed to safeguard the health of your endocrine glands. As the diseases of ageing take years to develop, you would be wise to initiate your anti-ageing program well before any of these diseases set in. I advise my patients to commence their programs from their mid-30s onwards, and in the rest of this book you will come to understand why this is so.

These are the health challenges that await you. Maintaining optimal antioxidant defences and preventing the age-related decline in the hormones that promote youthful energy are the keys to *Eternal Health*. In this book you will discover the means for achieving this. You will also learn that cancer can be prevented if you take the necessary precautions. You will encounter the means for boosting your brain power and rejuvenating your memory by more than 10 years. You will be informed as to how you can maximise your sexual potency naturally. You will acquire the means for effective weight loss and the ability to overcome debilitating fatigue while enhancing your energy and vitality. You will learn how to optimise your digestive process and maximise the detoxifying capabilities of your liver. We will tackle the thorny issue of Hormone Replacement Therapy (HRT) and all the problems that this difficult time engenders. Finally, you will be provided with all the new tests and anti-ageing protocols that assess all the parameters of ageing such as the effects of free-radicals on your mitochondria and your anti-ageing hormone levels. This is the medicine of the future. This is the medicine that utilises scientific methods for evaluating health and wellness rather than outdated forms of medical testing that inform you how diseased your body is.

By following the principles outlined in this book, you will be able to develop an action plan that you can utilise to dramatically improve your journey through life. Ageing is not inevitable and unavoidable. You can become an active participant in the medicine of the new millennium.

Key Points To Remember

Premature ageing is caused by the following:
• The decline in anti-ageing hormones.
• The accumulation of free-radicals.

The secrets to *Eternal Health* lie in:
• Neutralising the effects of free-radicals.
• Restoring youthful levels of the anti-ageing hormones.

CHAPTER 2

The Anti-Ageing Hormones

The Anti-Ageing Hormones

*I*T IS NO COINCIDENCE THAT THE AGEING PROCESS CORRESPONDS with the decline in certain key hormones. All the features of ageing—which include the degeneration of muscles, organs and bodily functions, the decline in immune function, the decreased efficacy of digestion and energy utilisation and the consequent loss of vitality—run in tandem with a dwindling supply of hormones such as human growth hormone, DHEA, melatonin and thyroid hormone. Although we're not sure why these hormones suffer age-related decline, it is not out of the question to postulate that ageing may be attributed to these hormonal changes. It becomes logical to consider then that restoring these hormones to their youthful levels is precisely what is needed to reverse the ageing process. This is what the proponents of anti-ageing medicine are claiming, and, although the jury is still out on this theory, all the evidence indicates that this is exactly what we should be doing. So once you have done everything you can to make sure that your battery is generating all the power it can, you then have to turn your attention to the energy that drives your motor. The best place to start is with the anti-ageing supremo, the master of all anti-ageing hormones— human growth hormone (HGH).

Human Growth Hormone (HGH)

The potency of this hormone is so profound that some scientists even propose that we need look no further than HGH for the cause of ageing. Recently a group of researchers at North Dakota State University were able to prolong the lives of mice, simply by administering a minuscule amount of growth hormone (1). Admittedly, we are not laboratory animals, but when evidence such as this stares us in the face, we need to pay attention. A significant number of interested physicians have been doing just that, and experiments have confirmed that HGH has enormous rejuvenating powers. HGH can reverse the biological clock almost on its own, which is why it is justifiably considered the hormone that promises the real 'fountain of youth'.

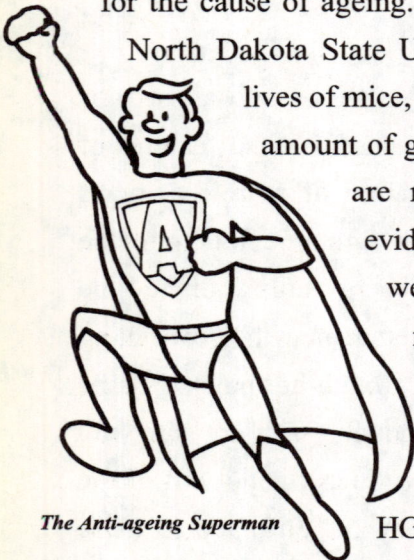

The Anti-ageing Superman

HGH is produced in your pituitary gland, which is located in the centre of your brain near the hypothalamus (Figure 3). The hypothalamus controls the production of HGH by means of two hormones: growth hormone releasing hormone (GHRH), which stimulates HGH release; and somatostatin, which blocks the output of HGH from your pituitary. Some claim that an imbalance between GHRH and somatostatin leads to the decline of HGH with age.

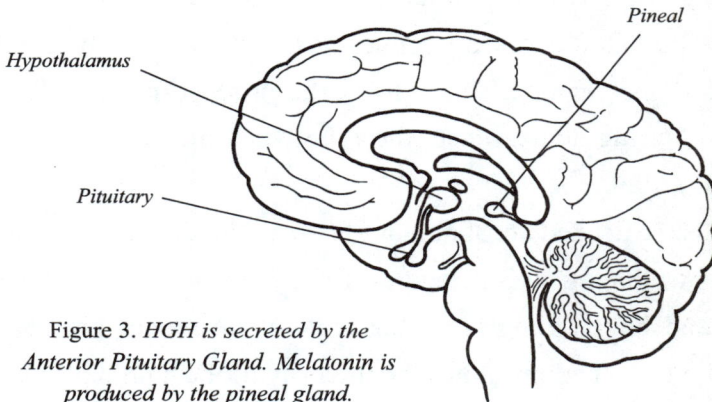

Pineal

Hypothalamus

Pituitary

Figure 3. *HGH is secreted by the Anterior Pituitary Gland. Melatonin is produced by the pineal gland.*

Once HGH is secreted by your pituitary it travels to your liver and other parts of your body where a substance called insulin-like growth factor 1 (IGF-1) is formed. IGF-1 is a partner to HGH as it performs its functions around the body. HGH hits its peak in adolescence, the period during which most bone growth occurs. After the age of 20, growth hormone production falls by 15 per cent per decade. This means that a 60-year-old secretes 25 per cent of the HGH produced by a 25-year-old. HGH is secreted in bursts during the day, but its prime activity takes place during the early hours of deep sleep. It is what HGH does that is so vital.

The Functions Of HGH

HGH stimulates the growth of bone, cartilage and connective tissue. Your bones become longer and stronger due to the effects of HGH. HGH builds protein, breaks down fat and makes glucose readily available for all the cells of your body. These are all the essential nutrients that your body needs to thrive and mature. This is why the production of HGH is so high during adolescence, the time when maximum growth occurs.

HGH is needed throughout life to maintain physical and mental wellbeing. HGH regulates body fat, increases muscle mass and bone strength, assists with tissue repair, preserves brain function and promotes the integrity of the hair, nails, skin and all the vital organs. Once HGH declines, everything tends to drop along with it. The body droops, the skin starts to sag, flab accumulates and muscle mass shrinks and becomes weaker. Hands grow softer and so does the penis, losing its former glory as it decreases in size. The decline in mental function and the deterioration in sleep patterns may also be related to changes in HGH production. This is the fate that awaits all of us as we grow older. However, we don't have to succumb to the consequences of diminished levels of HGH. These developments can be prevented if we become proactive about maintaining effective levels of HGH.

The Benefits Of HGH

Dr Daniel Rudman was the first to show the world how beneficial HGH therapy could be. In 1990, he administered HGH injections to 12 elderly men, aged 61 to 81 (2). To the delight of Dr Rudman and the participants in his experiment, impressive changes took place. There was an 8.8 per cent increase in muscle mass and a 14.4 per cent decrease in fat mass. Their bone density increased, their skins became thicker and their livers and spleens increased in size to the tune of a phenomenal 20 per cent. Unfortunately these changes were not sustained when the treatment was terminated. Three months after cessation of HGH therapy, the changes in muscle and fat mass reverted to their pre-treatment status. The initial improvements in bone density did not persist.

We have come a long way since those early days. From 1994 through to 1996 Drs Chein and Terry performed extensive trials on 800 patients using HGH therapy at the Palm Springs Life Extension Institute in the USA. What they did was administer HGH in doses that resembled the body's natural rhythm of HGH production. They found that over 80 per cent of the patients experienced enhanced energy levels, 88 per cent demonstrated improvement in muscle strength, 72 per cent reported significant fat loss, 75 per cent enjoyed increased sexual potency, and 70 per cent noted that their skin texture had thickened and their wrinkles had disappeared. A significant number also developed a more positive outlook on life and improved emotional stability.

This study was considered a landmark demonstration of the potent effects that HGH has on a diverse range of bodily functions. Since that time a number of studies have revealed how HGH therapy is able to improve the function of virtually every organ in the body.

HGH: The Most Powerful Antioxidant

One of the major causes of age-related cellular degeneration is the accumulation of free-radicals. To a certain extent these can be restrained by antioxidants. However, what free-radicals also do is activate proteases, which are destructive enzymes that damage cell proteins and essential cellular structures. This is where HGH comes to the rescue. HGH can activate a defence force of protease inhibitors that prevent these destructive forces from being initiated. While antioxidants can only reduce cellular levels of free-radicals, HGH can actually prevent any of the harm that free-radicals may cause. In addition to this, HGH is able to provide the nutrients needed to repair and regenerate cellular structures, thereby promoting the healing and renewal of ageing cells. It's no wonder that HGH is now recognised as the ultimate anti-ageing hormone.

Cardiovascular Health

When HGH levels fall, the risk of dying from cardiovascular disease doubles. The decline in HGH increases the risk of blood clotting, atherosclerosis and elevated blood pressure. The bad fats, which include LDL and triglycerides (see the chapter, 'Nurturing the Heart') tend to build-up and blood vessel walls become rigid and undistensible. HGH therapy reverses all these trends by decreasing LDL, lowering blood pressure and reducing atherosclerosis so that blood vessels become supple and rejuvenated. Another event that occurs with ageing is the weakening of heart muscle, leading to shortness of breath and fluid retention as the heart begins to lose its ability to pump blood around the body. HGH treatment is able to turn all this around, replacing a failing heart with one that works effectively and efficiently (3).

Boosting The Immune System

One of the systems that weakens with age is the immune system. This is partly due to the disappearance of the thymus gland, which is considered to be one of the primary activators of the immune system. The thymus is responsible for the maturation of T-cells, which protect the body against infectious diseases. Without this immune boosting effect, older people find themselves more vulnerable to invading organisms and diseases such as cancer. Infectious ailments that would not trouble a younger person may be lethal to an older person with no thymus gland.

Research workers in Israel and America have shown that in mice, injections of HGH can regenerate a shrivelled thymus gland thereby reactivating T-cell function. Not only did these animals have an improved immune system, but they were also found to live longer than a control group of animals who did not receive HGH injections.

It is widely acknowledged that HGH boosts all the cell types of the immune system including T-cells; B-cells; natural killer cells, which are very powerful inhibitors of invading micro-organisms; and macrophages, which gobble up bacteria.

Promoting Fat Loss

A feature of ageing is the accumulation of abdominal fat, which is strongly correlated with an increased risk of heart disease, diabetes and stroke. In Chapter 9, which details strategies for effective weight loss, you will learn how this form of weight gain is related to the development of cellular resistance to the hormone insulin. When this type of metabolic problem occurs, fat is stored instead of used for energy. Obese people make less HGH, which is especially significant because research shows that six months of HGH therapy is able to reduce abdominal obesity by 30 per cent (4). HGH encourages the burning of fat and promotes the building of muscle tissue. When HGH is around, cells respond to insulin in the appropriate manner, leading to the proper utilisation of fats, sugars and amino acids. This means that our hearts, brains and muscles are fed with the nutrients they need, while fat cells are induced to break down their existing stores.

Preventing Osteoporosis

Losing bone mass is another serious consequence of ageing. Although HGH is purported to stimulate the activity of osteoblasts—bone cells that increase the formation of new bone—the evidence that HGH increases bone density is not conclusive. Some studies show gains in bone mineral density while others demonstrate the opposite (5). It appears that the duration of therapy may be an important factor for determining whether HGH offers an added advantage. One study that did have positive implications for future management combined HRT in the form of 17B-oestradiol with IGF-1 therapy in rats that had their ovaries removed. This therapy was shown to improve bone remodelling and bone mineral content, which offers a potential new option for the long-term treatment of post-menopausal osteoporosis (6).

Sexual Vitality

Diminished sexual potency is one of the unfortunate consequences of ageing. Inability to sustain erections is a common problem for men over the age of 75. Users of HGH report an increase in libido and sexual vitality. Some men report longer lasting erections and frequency of sexual encounters is noted to increase (7).

Emotions And The Brain

HGH improves sleep and elevates mood. With a better night's sleep more HGH is produced, which doubles the benefit. HGH relieves depression by raising the levels of endorphins in the brain—chemicals that are associated with pleasurable feelings. HGH-deficient adults typically become withdrawn, socially isolated and pessimistic. With the introduction of HGH, this picture undergoes a complete makeover and these adults become sociable, friendly and outgoing. This scenario is not unlike the characteristic changes that the aged go through. Maintaining HGH levels turns this bleak landscape into a much more attractive canvas.

HGH may reverse the degeneration of nerve function that occurs with ageing. It is the connection between nerves that forms the basis for learning and memory, and it is this neuronal interplay that disappears with age. HGH stimulates nerve growth factors in the brain which cause new neuronal connections to form.

HGH Against Cancer

By boosting the immune system, HGH increases the body's natural resistance to cancer. In cancers of the liver, uterus and bowel, IGF-1 is reduced. One of the criticisms levelled against HGH therapy is that since IGF-1 (the partner of HGH) is growth promoting, tampering with nature in this fashion is a risky business. To date there is no evidence that HGH or IGF-1 stimulate cancer growth. If this were true we would expect cancers to be rife at a time when IGF-1 production is high during the mid-20s. We know that this is not the case. Experiments on animals show that HGH limits the growth and spread of certain cancers rather than enhancing cancer development.

HGH And The Way You Look

If you want to combat all those external signs of ageing, HGH is the wonder potion for you. It will not only make you feel younger, but you will enjoy all the advantages of looking more youthful. Renowned Belgian endocrinologist, Dr Thierry Hertoghe, who has researched the benefits of HGH for many years, has demonstrated that HGH reduces sagging cheeks, removes skin wrinkling, and replaces all those droops and bulges (including cellulite) with a body that is far more trim and taught. Even thinning grey hair can be supplanted with hair growth that is thicker and more lustrous.

There is now a growing base of scientific evidence that substantiates HGH'S rightful place as the premier hormone for regeneration and rejuvenation. HGH increases muscle mass, improves physical strength, renews brain function, protects the heart, enhances the immune system and rekindles sexual energy, leading to a demonstrably better quality of life. The only problem left to address is how to preserve this 'elixir of youth', as the anti-ageing physicians have termed it.

Stimulating HGH Production

Ever since Dr Daniel Rudman demonstrated that there is a hormone with amazing powers of renewal and restoration, the race has been on to develop the perfect means to boost HGH production. The decline in HGH with age is not inevitable as the pituitary can be stimulated to produce youthful levels of HGH at any stage of life. However, as you get older, the pituitary does not release the same bursts of HGH that it did when you were younger. Here are the means of delivering HGH to the body so that youthful levels can be restored.

HGH Injections

Injections of HGH made from recombinant DNA are probably the most powerful way of achieving the desired outcome of HGH augmentation. This technique has become relatively refined in that by dividing daily doses, the injections produce nearly physiological levels of HGH. The aim is to generate the levels of HGH that are typical of a 35-year-old. Because the amount of HGH administered is very modest, the side-effects that were seen with higher doses of HGH, such as fluid retention and joint pains, have been eliminated. The downside is the cost that can amount to as much as 800 to 1,000 dollars per month. In Australia, HGH is very difficult to obtain because you have to show a gross deficiency in HGH production before you can legally acquire it for therapeutic purposes. In reality most older people will have an HGH deficiency. The good news is that there are natural ways of increasing HGH without resorting to injections.

The Secretagogues

These are substances that stimulate the hypothalamus and the pituitary to produce more HGH. Amino acid-based formulas have been found to be very effective in enhancing HGH production. Arginine, ornithine, glutamine and lysine, when taken individually or in combination, have been shown to boost HGH levels. While arginine and ornithine have to be taken before bedtime in large doses, glutamine administered in modest amounts can raise HGH levels quite considerably. Cashews, almonds, mung bean sprouts and oat flakes are rich sources of arginine and lysine, while glutamine is found in foods such as rolled oats and cottage cheese.

Other research workers have focused on the diminishing effects that IGF-1 has at a cellular level. They claim that with ageing, our cells become resistant to the normal stimulatory effects of IGF-1, and, with this in mind, they have incorporated specific plant compounds in a formulation that makes cellular receptors more responsive to IGF-1 stimulation. They have combined these substances with amino acid secretagogues and other nutrients, and have reported very impressive results in a book titled The Methuselah Factor. The benefits noted included increased energy, improved muscle strength, reduced body fat and greatly enhanced libido.

Amongst the new growth hormone releasing substances, gamma-aminobutyric acid is considered to be the secretagogue with the most promise. If you resource the internet you will uncover a multitude of HGH-promoting substances, all promising the ultimate delivery system. All of these develop-ments are very exciting, but before you rush out and buy the latest formulation, it is worthwhile considering the natural ways of boosting your body's production of HGH.

Boosting HGH Production Naturally

High intensity exercise such as weight training, sprinting and squash will raise your HGH levels. Doing a really strenuous workout that involves the muscles of your lower body will increase HGH levels even more.

A high protein diet, which can be obtained from vegetarian sources, will provide the essential nutrients for optimal HGH production. Soybeans, almonds, lentils, wild rice, sunflower seeds and spinach are good examples of protein-rich foods that are hormone enhancing. Supernutrients such as spirulina, colostrum and noni juice contain protein complexes that promote hormone balance and give HGH a genuine shot in the arm.

The problem is that our lifestyles lead to premature HGH decline. Chronic, unresolved stress and poor eating habits inhibit HGH release. Simple exercise, a healthy diet and regular meditation will assist you in maintaining HGH levels that allow you to be youthful, strong and robust.

The hormones oestrogen, progesterone, testosterone, DHEA and melatonin are HGH stimulants. Along with HGH, these decline with age. In the forthcoming chapters you will learn how you can maintain youthful levels of these other hormones. For anyone who is committed to a life of exuberance and vitality, preserving HGH is one of the essential keys to super health. You are about to discover the other elements.

DHEA

Together with HGH and melatonin, DHEA (dehydroep-iandrosterone) is considered to be the anti-ageing hormone with the most potential to restore youthful levels of health and vitality. There is even evidence to suggest that older people with higher levels of DHEAS (the form in which DHEA is predominantly found in the bloodstream) survive longer (8). DHEA increases energy, improves ability to cope with stress and promotes physical and psychological wellbeing. Conversely, a decline in DHEA has been associated with a number of age-related problems such as osteoporosis, heart disease, obesity, loss of muscle mass and cancer. DHEA reaches peak production by the age of 25, after which levels diminish. The greatest decline has occurred by the mid-50s. By the age of 70, concentrations are 20 per cent (men) and 30 per cent (women) of what they were between the ages of 20 and 30. The trick lies in finding a way to preserve those early adulthood levels of DHEA, or at least augmenting your supply if your levels are running low.

To get a handle on how to do this, you need to understand some of the basics of DHEA formation. DHEA is made in your adrenal glands along with a number of other hormones. You probably know about the hormone adrenaline, which makes your heart beat faster and gives you that tight feeling in your stomach when you feel nervous. This is the so-called 'fight or flight' response, and what adrenaline is doing is making your body ready to deal with an immediate threat. The adrenals, which are two small pea-shaped glands situated on top of your kidneys, are also concerned with your long-term wellbeing. They may be small in size, but their impact on your health is astronomical. These tiny structures produce certain key hormones that play a vital role in safeguarding your welfare and maintaining the homeostasis of your body.

If you look at Figure 4 you will notice that there are three principal pathways emanating from the basic building blocks of cholesterol and pregnenolone. Pathways 2 and 3 are the ones we are concerned about. You will notice that pathway 2 leads to cortisol, while DHEA and DHEAS are located on pathway 3 where they give rise to the male and female sex hormones testosterone and oestradiol, the latter being the major female hormone.

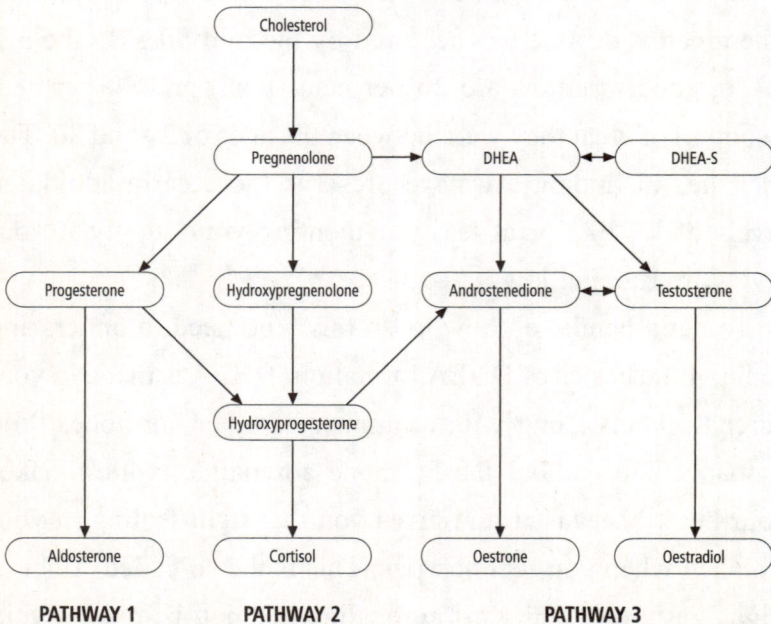

Figure 4.

Cortisol is released when the body has to deal with stress. As none of us are immune to this daily pleasure, the presence of cortisol in adequate amounts is essential for our survival. When we are stressed we need energy in the form of glucose to help us cope, and this is exactly what cortisol does. The trouble is, cortisol can become a touch overzealous in carrying out its daily duties, and, quite frankly, it doesn't give a damn where glucose comes from as long as there is a steady supply. So when glucose reserves are used up, the next place to obtain it is muscle. Cortisol will cause your muscles to release their protein so that glucose can be made. This leads to the gradual disappearance of muscle bulk. Cortisol also inhibits certain aspects of your immune system, causes your bones to lose their mineral content, and makes you put on weight. If you stop to consider what happens to the average individual after age 40, you will notice they accumulate fat around their waist, lose muscle on their arms and legs and become chubby in the face. These features result from excessive cortisol stimulation, and there are those who propose that ageing results from the body's response to chronic stress, with cortisol being the prime ageing hormone.

Stress is a feature of 20th century living that isn't helped by unhealthy lifestyle habits. Excessive coffee consumption, unresolved job conflicts, lack of exercise, poor sleep patterns and unsatisfying relationships vastly compound the litany of stressors that we encounter in our daily lives. Stress is unavoidable. It's the way we deal with it and reduce the effects of excessive cortisol stimulation that counts. This is what makes yoga, relaxation and/or meditation such essential components of any anti-ageing program.

If cortisol is the stress hormone, DHEA is the exact antithesis. DHEA stimulates your natural recuperative processes, allowing you to experience peace and tranquillity. Although it has never been proven, it is logical to imagine that when you are at peace your adrenals will produce more DHEA and less cortisol. This is one of the major challenges of any anti-ageing campaign, learning how to deal with stress so that the ratio of hormones produced by your adrenals favours DHEA.

If you return to Figure 4 you will notice that DHEA is made from pregnenolone, and that cholesterol is the building block for the synthesis of these two hormones. Pregnenolone is regarded as an anti-stress hormone in its own right and it has been noted to promote a sense of ease and peacefulness. To manufacture pregnenolone and DHEA you need the right nutrients, and, besides cholesterol, these include essential fatty acids and phospholipids. A diet that is rich in nuts, seeds, olives and fish will provide the right kind of fats for the development of the hormones that your body needs.

If you refer to Figure 4 you will notice that DHEA is converted to female sex hormones (oestradiol) and male sex hormones (testosterone). Males make 50 per cent of their sex hormones in the testes, the other half coming from adrenal DHEA. Most of the testosterone in women originates from DHEA, and in the chapter on sexual vitality you will learn how this impacts on female sexuality. What is equally important is that women depend on DHEA for their oestrogen. In the premenopausal phase, 75 per cent of oestrogen is synthesised from DHEA, with this figure rising to 100 per cent after menopause. This highlights the necessity for maintaining the adrenals in peak condition. Adrenals that are drained of energy will not provide sufficient amounts of DHEA for sex hormone production.

Research performed by Dr Samuel Yen over a 10-year period has revealed some of the numerous benefits of DHEA. Dr Yen found that six months of DHEA therapy in elderly folk increased their mobility, improved their sleep and boosted their immunity (9). He also noticed that men with high DHEA levels, without any supplementation, were less likely to die from heart disease, even if they smoked or had high cholesterol. Further studies confirmed that if DHEA levels were high, this was a surefire predictor of fitness, youthfulness and sexual vitality. Since that time there hasn't been a shortage of evidence testifying to the advantages of preserving the production lines of DHEA.

Charging The Immune System

DHEA operates in a similar way to HGH by boosting the immune system and increasing the immune cells that decline with age. One of the reasons that has been proposed for the deterioration of the immune system is the effect that free-radicals have in derailing any effective immune response, which intensifies with ageing. Like HGH, DHEA is considered a potent antioxidant with the ability to neutralise the effects of free-radicals, thereby offering considerable protection to the immune system. Research has demonstrated that old laboratory animals regain their youthful immunity once they are given DHEA. Such is the promise of DHEA that it has been used in AIDS sufferers with some effect. In a study carried out in the USA, DHEA was found to inhibit certain strains of the AIDS virus resistant to AZT (the potent anti-viral drug used in AIDS).

Cardiovascular Health

Heart disease is the leading cause of death in the elderly population so it's worthwhile pulling out all the stops to cut this dreaded scourge short in its tracks. Unfortunately the advantages seem to be more obvious in men who benefit from maintaining normal levels of DHEA. When DHEA levels drop, the chance of developing heart disease intensifies. In women, the relationship between DHEA and heart disease is a little more complex. Some studies show that DHEA lowers HDL (the good cholesterol) whereas others demonstrate that DHEA actually reduces serum triglycerides, cholesterol and LDL (the bad cholesterol), all of which are bad for the female heart (10,11). At this stage it's probably a line-ball decision as to whether DHEA is of benefit to female cardiovascular health. The safest thing to say is that we need more studies before any definite advice can be given.

DHEA Against Cancer

In animal experiments, DHEA has been found to suppress the growth of breast cancer. It also prevents cancer development in mice that have been exposed to a variety of chemical and viral agents. On the human front, there is a suggestion now that DHEA may inhibit the growth of bowel and prostate cancer. DHEA'S partner in this venture appears to be melatonin. Together they have the capacity to exert powerful anti-tumour effects. In his book Hormonal Health, Dr Michael Colgan, Director of the Colgan Institute of Nutritional Science in San Diego, indicates that both melatonin and DHEA protect against any stimulatory effects that oestrogen may have on breast tissue, thus making it possible for women to consider the possibility of going on HRT without the fear of initiating breast cancer. By preserving optimal levels of DHEA and melatonin, the risk of developing breast and other reproductive cancers may be eliminated.

DHEA, Alzheimer's Disease And Mental Health

DHEA has exciting potential for the prevention and treat-ment of Alzheimer's disease. With this tragic disease, the mental faculty that is eroded the most is memory. The area of the brain that is most responsible for memory is called the hippocampus, and DHEA has a protective effect on this region by inhibiting free-radical damage to hippocampal cells. In a fashion very similar to that of HGH, DHEA has been found to stimulate nerve growth as well as the connections between nerves. By enhancing brain function in such a manner, DHEA may play a vital role in reducing the destructive consequences of Alzheimer's disease.

DHEA has also been shown to reduce depression, improve sleep and promote emotional wellbeing.

DHEA And Osteoporosis

When menopause takes place, the adrenals become a major source for the hormones that look after female bones. If the adrenals are depleted they will not be able to provide sufficient DHEA for the synthesis of these hormones. Studies indicate that women with lower DHEA levels have a greater incidence of osteoporosis. DHEA increases bone mineral density and stimulates the formation of new bone, which has a much greater impact on bone health than the mere prevention of bone loss.

Managing Weight Gain

If you're looking for something to blame for the accumulation of fat, which typically occurs after the age of 40, look no further than the hormone insulin. Insulin likes to store fat, and once you start to put on weight it seems to encourage your fat cells to go into an even greater storage mode. Insulin doesn't like DHEA. When insulin levels go up less DHEA is produced, and the DHEA that is manufactured is more rapidly eliminated from your body. DHEA, on the other hand, reduces the fat storage effect that insulin has on your cells, so you will find it easier to lose fat and gain muscle, which is one of the keys to effective weight loss. Either you have to lose weight, which will reduce your insulin levels and in turn take the heat off DHEA, or you have to take supplementary DHEA if your levels are low, and wait for DHEA to restore your metabolism to fat-burning mode.

DHEA has also been found to effectively treat impotence, improve metabolic detoxification in the liver, and, most excitingly, increase IGF-1 levels(11). This is a strong testimony to the fact that the anti-ageing hormones work as a team, each reinforcing and activating the other. DHEA has a positive impact on a number of the pitfalls of ageing. We also know that DHEA production declines with age. The wisdom lies in finding ways to sustain the beneficial effects of DHEA.

Boosting DHEA Naturally

If you want to preserve DHEA production then you have to keep your adrenals as stress-free as possible. Dealing with unresolved emotional conflict, getting adequate sleep, relaxing several times during the day, and indulging in the pastimes that you enjoy the most may sound like reciting the obvious, but you'd be surprised how much these bare essentials lower your cortisol levels while enhancing the presence of DHEA. Certain nutrients play a central role in energising the adrenals. These include the following:

- *Vitamins A, B, C and E*
- *The minerals magnesium and zinc*
- *The amino acids tyrosine and phosphatidylserine*

The herbs ginseng and licorice are considered adrenal tonics. If you find that your energy is diminishing, you are putting on weight and your stress levels are mounting, it is highly likely that your adrenals are taking a pounding and it is time to reorganise your forces before the effects of elevated cortisol and insulin make serious inroads on your ageing process.

DHEA Supplements

The magical age of 40 is a good time to have your DHEA levels measured, along with all your other anti-ageing hormones. You can either have this done by means of a blood test or a salivary hormone assay. Salivary tests tend to be more accurate as they establish how much DHEA is actually active in your body, and an interesting way to go about this is to measure both DHEA and cortisol at various times of the day. This will tell you whether you are producing adequate amounts of DHEA or whether you are overwhelmed by stress and excess cortisol.

If you do need to replenish your supply of DHEA it is wise to do this as part of a general anti-ageing strategy that maintains the balance of all your anti-ageing hormones. Supplement dosages of DHEA range from 25 to 100mg, so it is probably best to commence at the lowest dose and have your levels measured regularly, together with the levels of the other hormones that are manufactured downstream from DHEA, like testosterone and oestradiol. DHEA has the power to restore youthful vitality. If you want to take full advantage of this anti-ageing tonic you have to ensure that all the players on your team are pulling their weight.

Melatonin

The hypothalamus and the pituitary are not the only glands that influence our hormones. Recent research indicates that ultimate control resides in the pineal, which secretes a hormone called melatonin. If you refer to Figure 3 you will notice that the pineal is located in close proximity to the hypothalamus and the pituitary. Hypothalamic output is modified by neurotransmitters coming from the brain, but its fate appears to depend on the outlay of melatonin produced by the pineal. As you can see in Figure 5, melatonin production steadily declines from adolescence onwards so that adults between the ages of 50 and 70 produce one tenth of the melatonin generated during this early period. One of the causes of the age-related decrease in HGH secretion is thought to result from this drop in melatonin. If you ever have the misfortune to need a CT scan, one of the observations that radiologists commonly make is to note the calcification of the pineal gland. This is a process that occurs with ageing and it means that your pineal is hardening up, resulting in the loss of melatonin-producing pineal cells. One way of removing these calcium deposits is by means of a substance called EDTA, which will be reviewed in Chapter 4.

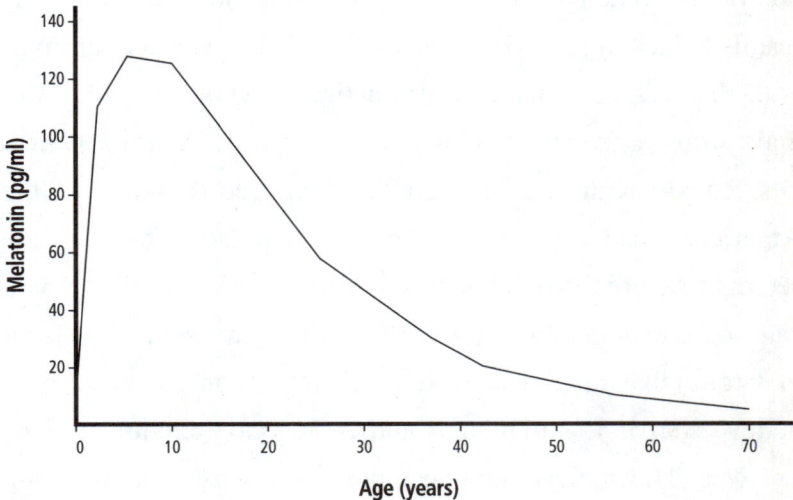

Figure 5.

EDTA is considered to be a very powerful chelator (remover) of calcium that has been deposited in unwanted places, along with any other heavy metal toxins.

Melatonin supervises metabolism at night and homeostasis during the day. Daily biological rhythms and sleep-wake cycles are determined by melatonin. All of life's major transformations such as puberty and the onset of the menstrual cycle are thought to be influenced by nature's biological clock in the form of melatonin. There is also evidence that demonstrates that melatonin can be harnessed to prolong life.

The most fascinating research on the manipulation of ageing by the administration of melatonin to laboratory animals has been performed by Italian immunologists. In 1988, a landmark study showed that when mice were given melatonin in their nightly drinking water their life-span increased by a substantial 20 per cent (12). What these research workers then went on to do was interchange pineals in young and old mice (13). The results achieved just what they expected. The younger animals with the older pineals aged dramatically while the older animals were rejuvenated with younger pineals. Herein, claims Drs Ronald Klatz and Robert Goldman, co-founders of the American Academy for Anti-Ageing Medicine, lies one of the secrets to eternal vitality. They are of the opinion that if you can somehow get the pineal to produce the same levels of melatonin that an adolescent does, then you can get the body to believe that it is still young and biological function will be renewed. They believe that once the pineal senses that the body is past its reproductive prime, production of melatonin is toned down and the ageing process is set in motion. Just as it is feasible for the pineal to trick the body, it is conceivable that by preserving youthful vitality you can persuade the pineal to maintain youthful levels of melatonin.

Like HGH and DHEA, melatonin has the ability to boost the immune system, fight cancer and nullify the effects of free-radicals.

The Immune System

Melatonin appears to augment the ability of HGH to regenerate the thymus gland. The mice that received melatonin in their drinking water enjoyed a longer life and acquired a greater resistance to disease. Their thymus glands were found to increase in weight, suggesting that they were making more T-cells that strengthened their immune systems.

Melatonin fortifies just about every aspect of the immune system. Immunoglobulins, CD4 cells and the powerful infection-fighting substances interferon and interleukin-2, are stimulated by the administration of melatonin. The time at which melatonin is taken is vitally important. If you supplement melatonin at night it will potentiate your immune system, however, if you take melatonin during the day it will become an immunosuppressant. Have you ever noticed that when you don't sleep very well for a period of time, you tend to come down with a virus more easily? This is because you need your sleep to produce adequate amounts of melatonin, and you need a good supply of melatonin to keep your immune system ticking over.

Melatonin Defeats Cancer

This is unquestionably the area of research that is yielding the most exciting discoveries, and, naturally, the most controversy. In an Italian newspaper, a recent headline informed the world that melatonin was found to be effective in the treatment of certain cancers for which no other medical treatment was considered useful. In some groundbreaking work, Dr Paolli Lissoni, was able to achieve what was thought to be the impossible (14). What he did was to demonstrate the positive effects of melatonin on patients with advanced cancer who were regarded as 'no-hopers'. These patients had already been given chemotherapy and they were given no more than six months to live. Lissoni gave these patients melatonin together with interleukin-2, which boosts the immune system. A survival time of longer than a year was achieved in no less than 43 per cent of the patients. This was seen as a monumental success as these kind of results had never been achieved before by conventional treatments.

When this information was released to the Italian community, it produced an outcry. Cancer sufferers on mass started to demand that they, too, receive the same treatment, and without doing any controlled trials, the medical establishment capitulated to the wishes of countless patients and started to utilise Lissoni's protocols. Sadly, the heroic achievements of Lissoni were not duplicated and many patients were left bitterly disappointed. This resulted in a vicious backlash against Lissoni's treatment, with many cancer specialists feeling vindicated for not jumping on the Lissoni bandwagon.

It's hard to know what to make of all this. Clearly, Lissoni achieved some kind of breakthrough and there are those doctors (myself included) who apply some of Lissoni's principles in the treatment of cancer patients with positive results. What we do need is more experimental work in this area, which is where the problem lies. Melatonin cannot be patented and this is probably why pharmaceutical companies are not bothering to initiate any clinical trials. No drug company stands to make huge amounts of money from any new discoveries involving melatonin, so there's no incentive for private investment. Other studies show that in laboratory animals, treatment with melatonin reduces breast cancer by a whopping 50 to 70 per cent. This has led other scientists to endorse melatonin as a possible means of dealing with other hormone-dependent cancers such as that of the prostate. At this stage it's premature to regard melatonin as the new cancer cure. Nevertheless, there is considerable promise in a remedy that does not have the toxic side-effects that chemotherapy engenders.

Melatonin: The Antioxidant

The free-radical barrage intensifies as we get older. Unfortunately this occurs at a time when our antioxidant defences are weakened and we are most vulnerable. The most destructive of all the free-radicals is the hydroxyl radical, an especially nasty piece of work. Because of its promiscuous nature,

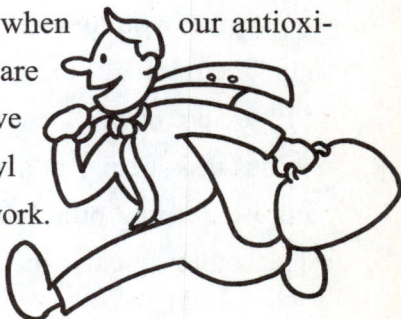

Am I glad I have a full bag of Melatonin

this toxic specimen is able to initiate a chain reaction that can have a profoundly destructive effect on the human body. Melatonin has been found to be a powerful neutraliser of hydroxyl radicals, far more so than any other antioxidant. Glutathione, vitamin C and vitamin E are thought to be extremely effective antioxidants, yet melatonin is the run-away winner when it comes to antioxidant fire-power. This hormone is twice as effective as vitamin E and five times more potent than glutathione. To illustrate how powerful melatonin is, rats that were given chow laden with cancer-promoting substances and melatonin, sustained 40 to 90 per cent less genetic damage than animals that were not given melatonin.

Melatonin Improves Sleep

Sleep disorders are so common that if I had a dollar for every patient that complained of insomnia I would be very wealthy by now. The problem is that there are no miracle potions. Drugs have side-effects: they can cause drowsiness in the morning and there is the long-term potential for addiction. As you age you might find it even more difficult to get a good night's sleep. When this happens you produce less melatonin, which gives you an even worse night's sleep, and round and round the mulberry bush you go.

If you are one of those unfortunate souls who finds sleep an onerous task, help is at hand. Melatonin could be referred to as nature's sleeping pill. Taking melatonin will allow you to fall asleep more quickly, increase the amount of time you spend asleep, and when you awake in the morning you will feel refreshed and ready to take on the challenges of the day. You need to take an average of 3mg of melatonin a couple of hours before you wish to go to sleep. By developing better patterns of sleep you will be safeguarding your production of hormones such as HGH and DHEA, and you now know how vital these hormones are.

Melatonin can also be taken to minimise jet lag. The best way to do this is to take melatonin shortly before bedtime in the new time zone and to continue doing this for the next three nights.

Melatonin Supplementation

Should you be taking melatonin? When should you start, and are there any harmful side-effects? With all the documented benefits that melatonin has to offer, and considering that melatonin has a controlling influence over your hormonal system and boosts HGH, you may be wise to at least entertain the notion of taking this substance. When you are in your 40s, it is a good time to get your melatonin levels checked. Melatonin is produced primarily at night when the pineal responds to darkness. Production peaks between midnight and 2am and then drops off until early morning. Salivary hormone assays would be the optimal way to measure your melatonin levels. Because of the daily fluctuation in melatonin, the best way to evaluate the presence of this hormone is by obtaining a sample in the morning and evening, which will detect the daytime baseline and nocturnal rise, respectively. If you are in your early 40s, a good dose to start off with is 1 to 2mg, taken on an empty stomach, an hour or two before you plan to retire. If your levels are very low, you can increase this dose up to 3mg. I advise patients not to increase their dose by more than 1mg per decade. It is wise to be cautious about melatonin. Taking too much of this hormone for too long a period of time can initiate an inflammatory process in your body. This means that your immune system becomes overactive and will start to attack your own body. For this reason melatonin is a no-no for those who suffer from auto-immune diseases such as rheumatoid arthritis and multiple sclerosis. Equally, certain cancers such as leukemia and lymphoma can be exacerbated by melatonin supplementation. For the under 35-year-olds, melatonin is not a good idea, neither is it a wise choice for pregnant women.

There are those foods that are melatonin boosting such as wild rice, tomatoes and ginger root, and a good time to have these would be during your evening meal. Melatonin is made from the amino acid tryptophan. By consuming more tryptophan-rich foods, which include soy products, almonds and peanuts, you will increase your natural production of melatonin.

Melatonin is another hormone that offers the 'elixir of eternal youth'. Although we still have a lot to discover about this wonderful hormone, those who ignore this substance are turning their backs on one of the potential marvels of nature.

Thyroid Hormone

Thyroid hormone is easily the most underrated and under-valued hormone in the anti-ageing scheme of things. It's probably not seen as being as sexy as HGH, melatonin or DHEA, but its contribution to health and vitality is just as important. I would say that at least half of my patients demonstrate some of the symptoms of thyroid hormone deficiency. Do you feel lethargic, sluggish and depressed? Do your hands and feet feel constantly cold? Are you struggling to lose weight no matter what diet you try? Are you suffering from increasing hair loss, diminishing libido and a general lack of motivation? If so, these are indications that your thyroid hormone is not doing the job it should, and you need to discover what you can do to rectify this metabolic imbalance. Aside from undergoing a very subtle decline with age, there are a number of factors that impede the normal daily activities of thyroid hormone.

The Function Of Thyroid Hormone

Thyroid hormone controls the metabolic activity of all our cells. When we talk about metabolism we are essentially talking about energy generation. What thyroid hormone does is stimulate our cells to use oxygen in order to create energy. This is what the basal metabolic rate (BMR) is all about. The BMR diminishes when thyroid hormone ceases to function adequately and this is when you will find that everything starts to slow down.

Thyroid hormone also facilitates protein synthesis, which allows for the manufacture of vital enzymes. Without sufficient enzymes, biochemical reactions within cells cannot take place. Proteins form part of the structure and transport functions that transpire in our cells. By activating these substances, thyroid hormone regulates the function of all the organs in our bodies. Thyroid hormone is responsible for controlling the rate of absorption of nutrients in the gastrointestinal tract, and is necessary for the secretion of the sex-activating hormones from the pituitary gland. Thyroid hormone is also paramount for normal bone growth as well as for the maturation of your nervous system. Your immune system, cholesterol and triglyceride levels are influenced by the presence of thyroid hormone. Diabetes, heart disease and osteoporosis are long-term consequences of the insufficient production of thyroid hormone. It's not difficult to appreciate then that when thyroid hormone ceases to do its thing, a lot can go wrong. Anti-ageing experts claim that low thyroid hormone undermines longevity, so it's pretty important that we understand how to prevent this from happening.

The Manufacture Of Thyroid Hormone

Thyroid hormone is made by the thyroid gland, which is situated at the front of your throat. Iodine and the amino acid tyrosine are two of the essential nutrients you need to manufacture thyroid hormone. The B vitamins are particularly important, especially vitamins B2, B6 and B12. Vitamins A, C and E are also key nutrients. Animal studies have shown that deficiencies of these vitamins results in inadequate production of thyroid hormone.

Thyroid hormone exists in your body in two forms: thyroxine, which is also called T4; and triiodothyronine, which is quite a mouthful, also called T3. T4 is converted into T3 primarily in your liver and kidneys, and it is T3 that is the predominant executor of thyroid hormone function in your body. To convert T4 to T3 you need certain nutrients such as zinc, selenium and the amino acid cysteine. The hormones melatonin and HGH impact on this conversion as well. Because absorption of all nutrients declines with age and hormones diminish, T3 is very commonly under-produced. It is therefore not surprising that fatigue, weakness, stiff joints and loss of memory, which are all symptoms of thyroid deficiency, are also manifestations of the ageing process. There is, however, another metabolic syndrome, which is not well recognised by the medical fraternity, that accounts for a large percentage of thyroid hormone problems.

Reverse T3 Dominance Syndrome

In case you think that this is some kind of sado-masochistic aberration, let me explain. Here's how the story goes. When your body converts T4 to T3 another tiny substance is formed called Reverse T3 (RT3). RT3 has a profound action on your metabolism by blocking the action of T3. RT3 makes you slow down and causes a drop in your body temperature. This drop in temperature lulls all the enzymes in your body into a state of inertia, and this is when you start to suffer from lethargy, irritability, fluid retention, low sex drive, decreased memory, low motivation and all the other features of thyroid hormone deficiency. Yet, you are not deficient in thyroid hormone. RT3 is simply taking over. In the normal course of events, T3 dominates and RT3 is no problem.

However, in a situation when stress is prolonged, the adrenal glands pump out excessive amounts of our old enemy cortisol. Cortisol inhibits the conversion of T4 to T3 and favours the conversion of T4 to RT3. If stress is unresolved and ongoing, a condition called Reverse T3 Dominance occurs and continues even after the stress abates and cortisol levels fall. This leads to a state of affairs that mimics thyroid hormone insufficiency. Apparently this syndrome is vastly under-diagnosed, with the incidence being about 20 per cent of the general population. Eighty per cent of these people who visit doctors complain of the aforementioned symptoms.

There are other factors that lead to Reverse T3 Dominance. These include zinc and selenium deficiency, which emphasises the importance of these two minerals, starvation, sleep deprivation, and a condition called Wilson's syndrome, which I will discuss shortly. The notion that starvation precipitates RT3 is an interesting point to consider for those who are of the opinion that prolonged fasting is the best way to lose weight. Even when the fast is terminated, RT3 will remain in the ascendancy, which means that metabolism will remain in first gear for a prolonged period of time and fat will be that much harder to shed.

Wilson's Syndrome

This is a condition that is more common in people whose ancestors survived famine such as the Irish, the Scots, the Welsh and the Russians. Also, it appears that about 80 per cent of sufferers are women. Typically the symptoms, which can include PMS, irregular periods, anxiety attacks, dry skin and constipation, as well as the other customary features of RT3 Dominance, tend to come on after a major stressful event. Another hallmark of this syndrome is persistently low body temperature. In fact, this is one of the ways to diagnose this condition. You need to take your temperature at least three times a day for three days and then average it out. Normally your average will be 37 degrees. If the average is 35 to 36 degrees and you have some of the above mentioned symptoms, then it is highly likely that you have Wilson's syndrome.

Thyroid Function Tests

In order to find out whether you have a thyroid hormone problem you need to have tests that cover all the parameters of thyroid hormone function. This includes T4, T3, RT3, basal body temperature and TSH (thyroid stimulating hormone that comes from the pituitary). If your ratio of T3 to RT3 is less than 10 to one, if you have a low temperature and the other symptoms of a metabolism that has slowed down, then you need to commence some form of therapy that restores T3 to its normal function.

Thyroid Hormone Supplementation

As well as addressing all the causal factors—and this involves dealing appropriately with stress, optimising the function of your liver where T3 is made, and making sure that you have adequate resources of selenium and zinc—you might need to take some form of thyroid hormone supplement. This is where the difficulty arises as the standard drug treatment for thyroid hormone insufficiency is made up of only T4 and not T3, despite the fact that it is usually with T3 that the problem resides. Fortunately alternatives are available, either in the form of Time Release T3 Therapy or desiccated thyroid extract, which is made up of a combination of T3 and T4. These treatments will allow you to bring your T4 and T3 into optimal balance, restoring your metabolism to its usual efficiency.

Key Points To Remember

The anti-ageing hormones that promote vitality and well-being include:

- HGH
- DHEA
- Melatonin
- Thyroid hormone

Collectively these:

- Boost the immune system.
- Enhance the body's antioxidant defences.
- Increase libido and sexual vitality.

- Reduce the diseases of ageing such as osteoporosis, heart disease, Alzheimer's disease and cancer.
- Improve ability to cope with stress.
- Control the basal metabolic rate.
- Rectify poor sleep patterns.
- Increase muscle mass and reduce body fat.
- Prolong life in laboratory animals.
- Elevate mood and promote a feeling of general wellbeing.

The Gut and Liver - A Solid Foundation

THREE

The Gut and Liver

A Solid Foundation

*T*HE GUT DIGESTS AND ASSIMILATES WHILE THE LIVER DETOXIFIES. In a nutshell, this is what these organs have to do if you want to give yourself a fighting chance of beating all the metabolic challenges that life is going to throw your way. If you can safeguard these fundamental processes then you will provide a solid foundation upon which you can build your anti-ageing program. Unfortunately my clinical experience indicates that precious few have a healthy gut or a fully functioning liver. We live in an age where gastrointestinal disorders are rife and this does not augur well for healthy ageing. A recent study indicates that over a three-month period, over 70 per cent of households experience one or more gastrointestinal symptoms. Why is it that we have such woeful digestive systems? Is there some sort of secret to preserving healthy digestive function? On the contrary, it's really very simple. What you have to do is take the time to focus on key digestive processes. Just as eating can be a delightfully enjoyable pastime if you allow yourself to savour each mouthful, digestion can be maintained in its most pristine form if you take the appropriate care. To get a sense of how much attention you need to devote to restoring optimal gut health, complete the following symptom questionnaire.

Evaluate your response to the following symptoms according to this rating scale:

0 = never, 1 = twice a week, 2 = three to six times a week, 3 = daily or several times per day.

- Excessive burping
- Offensive breath
- Sores in corner of mouth
- Bloating
- Excessive passage of gas
- Heartburn and indigestion
- Alternating diarrhoea and constipation
- Dry flaky skin and brittle hair
- Poorly formed stools
- Anal itching

Scores:

0-5:   You have an excellent digestive system

6-10:   Not bad, but you could do with a tune up

11-16: You need to take care, you are heading into trouble.

17-23: A poor digestive process, you need a comprehensive gut evaluation.

24-30: See your health care practitioner immediately before your insides implode.

I would say that a vast majority of my patients survive in the 17-and-over category. What this does is allow microbes and toxins that are potentially lethal to establish a cosy little home for themselves in the gut. Your bowel then has to furiously rally its forces to protect you from these dangerous intruders. This prevents digestion and assimilation from proceeding at a relaxed and efficient pace. If the lining of the bowel is breached by these organisms, the liver will have to deal with all these toxins. If the liver's detoxification pathways become overloaded, free-radicals will multiply. The consequence is accelerated ageing in all its various guises. This is why naturopathic physicians have been extolling the virtues of a healthy gut since time immemorial. Maybe the moment has arrived for us to take notice. If you want to maintain your digestive process in mint condition there are four principal factors you need to be aware of:

- Digestive enzymes
- A healthy gut ecology
- Eating the foods that are appropriate for you
- Maintaining the lining of your gut wall

Digestive Enzymes

These are fundamental to the digestive process and you'd be shocked at how often these bare essentials are found to be lacking. The stomach secretes hydrochloric acid and an enzyme called pepsinogen, which go about their business of digesting protein, as well as facilitating the absorption of certain vitamins such as vitamin B12. Hydrochloric acid also acts to kill bacteria and parasites. Having an adequate supply of hydrochloric acid is a prerequisite for optimal digestion and assimilation to occur. Without it the digestive process starts to break down.

A significant proportion of adults, particularly those over the age of 50, do not produce enough hydrochloric acid. This leads to deficiencies in protein, the most vital of nutrients, and vitamin B12, a nutrient that every cell of your body needs to perform basic metabolic functions. Symptoms such as burping, indigestion, bad breath and partial loss of taste suggest that you are not secreting enough hydrochloric acid. How often do you go to the doctor with some sort of digestive complaint, and what do you get? Some form of medication that suppresses your production of hydrochloric acid, which ultimately weakens your digestive process. Rather than take an antacid, more often than not you need something that will enhance the presence of this essential digestive substance.

There are a number of reasons for having an inadequate supply of hydrochloric acid. Stress, overeating and diets that don't provide the right nutrients, especially those that are deficient in zinc, ultimately compromise hydrochloric acid production. Helicobacter pylori, which is now regarded as the primary cause of stomach ulcers, can also drain your resources of hydrochloric acid. The cells of your stomach go into overdrive in an attempt to rid you of this organism and eventually your reserves of hydrochloric acid become depleted. Lacto-bacillus acidophilus, which is regarded as one of the friendly intestinal bacteria, and vitamin C have been found to be effective in combating heli-cobacter pylori, so if you prefer to pass on the conventional antibi-otic treatment for this organism, natural alternatives are available.

If I suspect that a deficiency of hydrochloric acid is the problem behind a digestive complaint, then what I recommend is a daily glass of water with a freshly squeezed lemon. This gets the digestive juices flowing very efficiently. For those who enjoy some of the traditional remedies, apple cider vinegar is another digestive stimulant.

The other essential component of the digestive process is the pancreatic enzymes. These have a huge role to play as they are involved in the digestion of fats, carbohydrates and proteins. Symptoms that result from deficiencies of pancreatic enzymes include bloating, excessive gas, fatigue and poorly formed stools that contain lots of undigested material. In his book Food Enzymes For Health And Longevity, Dr Edward Howell claims that we eat far too much cooked food, which gives the pancreas too much work to do. Evidence shows that the human pancreas is one of the heaviest in the animal kingdom. Raw food provides a rich source of enzymes that assist in the digestive process. Cooked food is lacking in enzymes and provides less of the vital nutrition that the pancreas needs to function. This type of diet, which is also usually high in sugar and fat, disturbs the acid-base balance of the gut in favour of a more acidic environment. Ultimately pancreatic enzyme secretion will diminish in an attempt to deal with this problem.

Supplemental digestive enzymes are usually the best way to treat pancreatic enzyme deficiency. Plant-derived products contain the full spectrum of pancreatic enzymes and these have been found to be the most effective.

A Healthy Gut Ecology

Your digestive juices need a healthy internal environment in which they can thrive. This is provided by what is loosely termed 'the friendly bacteria', as well as a good dose of fibre. There are a host of micro-organisms residing in your gut. The friendly bacteria are those that live in harmony with your gut and assist with digestion and absorption of nutrients. Examples include species such as acidophilus and bifidobacteria. A second group are called the commensals. These micro-organisms simply sit on the fence watching the action. They do neither harm nor good and are comprised of the E.coli and streptococci species. A third family of bacteria are the pathogens. These are the ones you have to be wary of as they are capable of damaging the lining of your intestinal tract and producing toxins that may be absorbed into your bloodstream. Among these bacteria are the clostridia, salmonella and campylobacter species.

Candida albicans is a very interesting type of micro-organism. Mostly it is a commensal, idly going about its daily activities along with the rest of the microbes in your gut. There

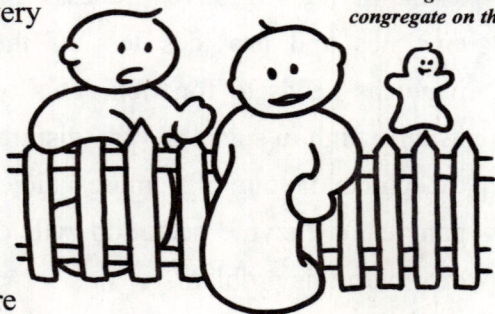

Some germs like to congregate on the fence

is a theory that it becomes a source of bother when it mutates into its pathological fungal form. Then it is able to burrow through the lining of the gut wall and give off toxins that cause all sorts of damage to a variety of systems around the body.

I want to emphasise that this is not a proven scientific fact. Nevertheless, I utilise the anti-candida program in my practice and find it to be useful in treating certain types of chronic conditions such as acne, eczema and irritable bowel syndrome. I have found a yeast and sugar-free diet that contains lacto-bacillus acidophilus, bifidus and bulgaricus bacteria, together with herbal formulations comprising agents such as olive leaf concentrate, grapefruit seed and pau d'arco to be most effective.

If you want to prevent all the chronic illnesses associated with ageing such as arthritis, dementia, heart disease and the proliferation of free-radical toxins, which are associated with the development of cancer, then you have to encourage the friendly bacteria to flourish. This will discourage the growth of unfavourable organisms and reduce the secretion and absorption of harmful microbial poisons into the bloodstream.

Lactobacilli, which appear to head the family of benevolent organisms, have other beneficial functions to perform. They synthesise B vitamins and lower cholesterol levels. Most importantly they convert soluble fibre to butyrate, which is the primary fuel for the cells lining the colon. This is reputed to be an anti-cancer agent that serves to prevent the development of colon cancer and other cancers.

Having adequate fibre helps to maintain a healthy population of friendly bacteria. Vegetarians who consume fibre-rich diets have been found to have a high percentage of lactobacilli in their stools and a lower quota of pathogenic bacteria such as clostridia. A high-fibre diet is very cancer protective as it promotes the elimination of harmful hormones and other undesirable toxins by establishing an optimal transit time and complete daily evacuations.

Dietary fibre is found in two forms, soluble and insoluble. Soluble fibre dissolves in water and stimulates the growth of favourable bacteria. Examples include apples, carrots, oat bran and psyllium husks. Wheat bran, brown rice, lentils, asparagus and flaxseed are high in insoluble fibre. These foods increase stool bulk and speed up transit time. They protect against pathogenic organisms by ensuring that they are expelled from the body.

A substance that is becoming extremely popular as an enhancer of gut health is bovine colostrum. Colostrum is the first substance to be secreted in breast milk, and the bovine form is derived from the initial food produced by the cow for the calf. It is a white powder that contains powerful immune boosting nutrients that neutralise toxins and counter the establishment of any foreign organisms in your gut. It contains little milk. Colostrum also has certain constituents that bind to harmful bowel bacteria such as helicobacter pylori, thereby preventing their attachment to the intestinal mucosa. Colostrum has been used in trials to treat both rheumatoid arthritis and osteoarthritis and the results to date are very promising (2).

To discover whether your gut ecology is in good shape you need to have a test called the Comprehensive Digestive Stool Analysis (CDSA). The CDSA is the closest you can get to evaluating the balance of your gut flora. It reveals whether you have a healthy level of lactobacilli species or an overgrowth of the pathogenic bacteria. It also provides some indication as to the performance of your digestive enzymes and the presence of favourable metabolic substances in your gut. The CDSA is performed by laboratories mentioned at the back of this book. It is not a component of the routine stool testing carried out by laboratories in Australia. If you have gut problems or would like to have this type of assessment as part of your anti-ageing program, a CDSA can provide you with valuable information.

Eating The Right Foods

Food allergies or intolerance is a very common problem that can lead to a multitude of systemic conditions including those that are synonymous with premature ageing such as arthritis, fatigue, inflammation of the arteries, heart disease and even diminished sex drive. It is necessary to indicate that, once again, this is conjecture and not proven scientific fact. We don't know for sure that foods cause all these problems, nor do we understand how they actually arise. This is why we like to use the term 'intolerance', which means some foods or the constituents thereof cause negative reactions in the gut and possibly the rest of the body, but we are not certain as to what the mechanisms are for this type of effect. However, this hasn't stopped countless experts from proposing various hypotheses. The most plausible explanation to date suggests that when you are exposed to a substance that causes you to react in an adverse fashion, inflammatory reactions and free-radical toxins are elicited. These reactions are designed to neutralise the effects of the foreign substances invading your body. Inadvertently, your own bodily tissue gets caught in the crossfire, which leads to the development of such chronic conditions as arthritis, fatigue and inflammatory bowel diseases.

Unfortunately the time delay between the development of symptoms and the ingestion of the offending substances can be protracted, so it's not always possible to identify the culprit. The truth is in there, it's just a matter of donning your best Sherlock Holmes hat. One helpful clue is that the food that causes you the most trouble is paradoxically the substance you crave the most. This is because your body maladapts to the substance in question to prevent withdrawal symptoms, somewhat like an addiction. An example of this is the child who initially develops colic in response to cows milk, then goes on to develop asthma, and finally suffers from headaches, depression and arthritis in adult life. All the while it is milk that is causing the problem, yet this unhappy individual may have a real attachment to consuming dairy products. The real challenge is giving up this class of foods, as, initially, the body will not relinquish this pattern of behaviour easily.

Once you have discovered the cause of your problem you will have to set about eliminating the offending foods from your diet. Dr Peter D'adamo in his now famous Eat Right 4 Your Blood Type diet, has made it simple for us by indicating that certain blood types are suited to certain diets. If your blood group is type O you should eat meat and avoid wheat. Blood type As are suited to a vegetarian lifestyle. Type Bs can vary their diets to include vegetable and animal protein, and they are the only blood type that does well with dairy products.

Type ABs should be on the lookout for problems emanating from dairy and wheat consumption. Although this type of approach places everyone on the planet into four basic categories, and not everyone will respond to such an approach, I have found the use of the blood-type diet to be effective in certain cases.

An interesting question is: why do so many people suffer with food intolerance if eating is such a natural and enjoyable part of life? The sense I make out of it is that our digestive processes are not used to the consumption of refined and processed foods, and this problem will probably get worse with the production of genetically engineered substances. For this reason I encourage my patients to eat organically grown fruits and vegetables to avoid this kind of contamination.

Maintaining The Lining
Of Your Gut Wall

If you have any chronic illness associated with food intolerance, chances are you also have increased intestinal permeability or what is termed 'the leaky gut syndrome'. The lining of our gut forms a barrier between the internal environment and the rest of our body. If we are over-exposed to toxic substances and the supports for this intestinal membrane are weak, then it is possible for this barrier to be penetrated and toxins can pass into the bloodstream. This results in chronic disease that is pretty much along the same lines as food intolerance. In fact the two are inextricably linked.

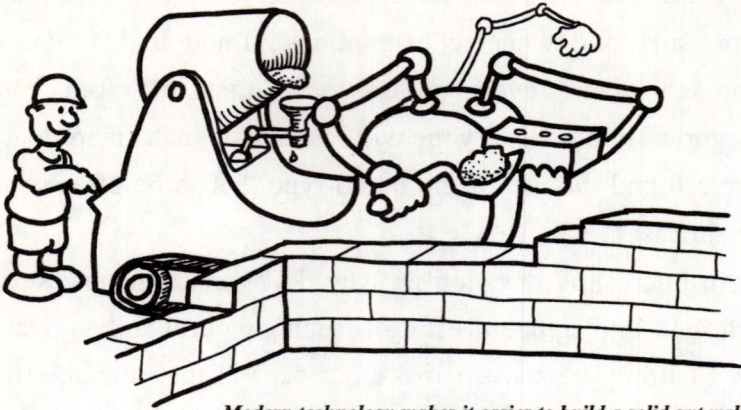

Modern technology makes it easier to build a solid gut wall

There is a test you can take to evaluate whether you have the leaky gut syndrome. The lactulose/mannitol test assesses the presence of these substances in your urine. Normally you do not absorb large molecules like lactulose, which is a type of sugar. However, if you have a leaky gut it is possible. Mannitol, which is a small sugar, should be absorbed without any problem. If you find that you do have abnormalities based on the results of this test, then what you would need to do is undertake a gut repair program that is designed to heal the damage done to the lining of your bowel so that you no longer absorb any of the toxic substances that adversely affect your health. This program involves the avoidance of common offending foods as well as the incorporation of certain nutrients in your diet that can restore the normal function of the cells of your gut. These agents include vitamins A, C, E, the B vitamin pantothenic acid, the mineral zinc and the amino acid glutamine, which provides fuel for the intestinal cells.

Providing your bowel with the best nourishment certainly pays dividends. If you don't you will find yourself at the mercy of countless toxins and free-radicals that dramatically accelerate the ageing process. Then you will have to rely on the resources of your liver to rescue you.

The Liver

One of the principal functions of the liver is to detoxify every chemical the body encounters by transforming them into readily excretable substances that can be eliminated by the body. This detoxification process involves a number of complex biochemical pathways, and, to tell you the honest truth, there is a lot we don't understand about the intricacies of this undertaking. There are indications that if you experience tiredness, irritability and inappropriate anger, then your liver is not dealing adequately with its toxic load. Easy bruising, bleeding tendencies in the gums and nose and reddened skin around the palms are clear signs that your liver is in trouble.

Even though we do not yet have a complete handle on how the liver works, I advise all of my patients, especially those with the above features, to eat lots of garlic, onions, nuts, seeds and cruciferous vegetables like cabbage, cauliflower and broccoli. These foods are thought to nourish the biochemical pathways that implement detoxification. I also suggest that they supplement their diets with the B group vitamins as well as vitamins A, C and E for additional liver support. There is a nutrient called S-adenosylmethionine (SAMe), which is now regarded as the number one enhancer of liver detoxification. It is being heralded in some quarters as a 'multi-functional supernutrient'. Studies show that SAMe increases the amino acid glutathione, another nutrient implicated in liver function, and together these two demonstrate a lot of promise in restoring the detoxification process. SAMe has been found to reduce the risk of liver cancer in individuals whose livers have been damaged by alcohol, toxins and diseases such as hepatitis. In mice, SAMe protects the liver from the lethal effects of acetaminophen.

The liver is a very resilient organ with a high capacity to regenerate. Unfortunately we seem to be finding a way to stretch the resources of our livers to the limit with a steady bombardment of chemicals, pollutants and drugs. My counsel is, until we have the final word on the exact biochemical workings of the liver, do all you can to keep this vital organ in perfect condition.

Key Points To Remember

These are the signs of poor digestion:

• Burping

• Bloating

• Bad breath

• Excessive passage of gas

Optimal digestion depends on:

• Digestive enzymes

• A healthy gut ecology

• The integrity of the gut wall

• Eating the right foods

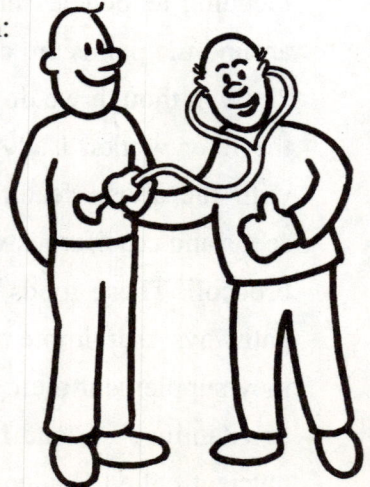

That sounds like an excellent liver!

Poor liver detoxification may lead to:

- Tiredness
- Irritability
- Inappropriate anger

Foods and nutrients that enhance liver detoxification include:

- Garlic
- Cruciferous vegetables
- S-adenosylmethionine (SAMe)
- Glutathione
- Vitamins A, B complex, C and E

CHAPTER 4

Nurturing The Heart

Nurturing
The Heart

THE COMPLEXION OF CARDIOVASCULAR HEALTH HAS UNDERGONE A major facelift in recent times. No longer does it suffice to entertain the traditional risk factors, including smoking, family history, cholesterol and blood pressure, and think that by having these under control you are doing all that you need to do to look after your heart. It's a whole new world out there. If you want to stay in touch with current developments there is a lot more for you to discover. Oxidised cholesterol, inflammation, insulin resistance, homocysteine, lipoprotein(a) and fibrinogen are currently being recognised by medical science as the primary enemies of the ongoing health of your heart. These are terms that you need to become familiar with if you want to position yourself at the forefront of 21st century cardiovascular health. Rest assured that these new processes are very easy to understand, and, more importantly, even easier to prevent if you take all the necessary steps. The most exciting fact of all is that there are drug-free methods you can employ to optimise the health of your heart, thereby preventing any of the above mentioned processes from impacting on your cardiovascular system.

Considering that heart disease is the number one killer of the baby boomer generation, it is vital that you know all there is to know about the health of your heart. This revolution in the way we view cardiovascular health has transpired partly because of some recent research findings that have cast serious doubt on the validity of the cholesterol theory of heart disease. "What!" I can hear you saying, "Does this mean that I won't have to worry about my cholesterol levels any more and I can tuck into that juicy steak?" Well, not exactly, but let's take a look at the facts to see how the cholesterol theory has stood up under the scrutiny of scientific testing.

One protracted study done in a small Dutch town called Zutphen, set out to discover exactly what sort of impact cholesterol actually has on the incidence of heart attacks (1). After five years, no association was found between cholesterol and death due to myocardial infarction (heart attack). What researchers did find most significant however, was the high level of a specific antioxidant called quercetin in those townsfolk who had the least incidence of myocardial infarcts. When this fact became glaringly obvious, the cholesterol study was abandoned for one that assessed the benefits of antioxidants on the prevention of heart disease. These revelations set the stage for further studies concerning the cholesterol hypothesis.

In 1991, a Finnish study found that business executives who were placed on a low-cholesterol diet were more than twice as likely to succumb to heart disease as compared with individuals who remained on a normal diet (2). Other studies have shown that folk over the age of 75 who have moderately elevated cholesterol levels do better with regard to heart disease than those with normal cholesterol levels. Further studies indicate that at least a third of the individuals who suffer from heart attacks have, would you believe, normal cholesterol levels.

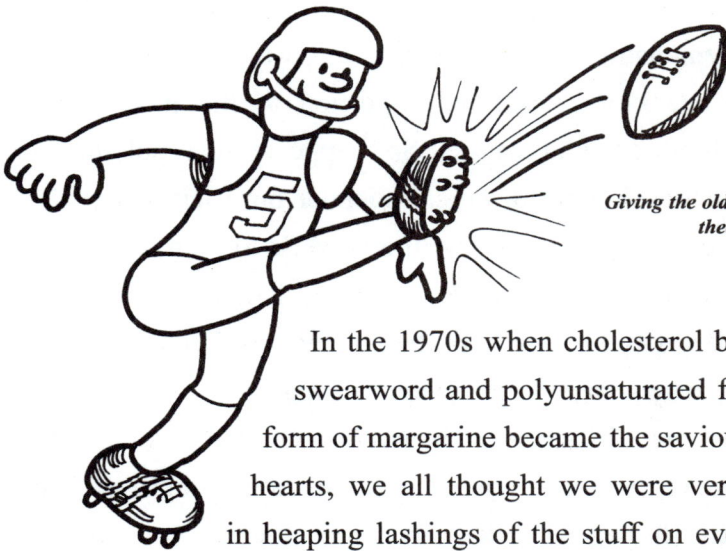

Giving the old cholesterol theory the boot

In the 1970s when cholesterol became a swearword and polyunsaturated fat in the form of margarine became the saviour of our hearts, we all thought we were very clever in heaping lashings of the stuff on every slice of bread that passed through our alimentary tracts. The polyunsaturated fat diet was welcomed as 'the prudent diet', and when this type of culinary recommendation was found to reduce cholesterol by a massive 25 per cent, scientists at that time were patting themselves on the back. Needless to say the companies that were manufacturing margarine made bundles of money on the back of huge advertising campaigns. Eggs and butter became identified as the villains and were relegated to the nutritional scrap heap. Of course every theory demands some sort of scientific backup and this is exactly what researchers at the time set out to do, confident that they would substantiate what they thought was a foregone conclusion.

What they discovered was an unmitigated disaster. Study after study confirmed the opposite of what they had hoped for. The prudent diet, high in polyunsaturated fat, offered no advantage in preventing heart disease. In fact, what these studies demonstrated quite conclusively, was that deaths due to heart attack increased in proportion to the increase in polyunsaturated fats in the diet. So it appeared that polyunsaturates and low cholesterol weren't so much our friends after all. It took the intelligentsia of the time a while to realise that the polyunsaturated vegetable oils had been denuded of antioxidants, and it was this lack of protection that resulted in some of the damage these type of fats were causing.

Later it was discovered that polyunsaturated fats actually set in motion a process called inflammation, which, as you will learn shortly, is extremely damaging to your blood vessels. In fact, oxidation and inflammation are now widely considered to be the major instigators of heart disease and it is really the extent of these two processes in your body that need to be evaluated if you really want to know whether you are at risk of sustaining any form of cardiovascular disease. Before we move on to discuss these exciting new perspectives, I need to say a few more words about cholesterol.

This poor substance has become so vilified that it is hard to imagine that it has any redeeming characteristics. You would be surprised to discover that cholesterol is an antioxidant in its own right, and it is located in cell walls where it protects cell membranes. If you refer back to Figure 4 in Chapter 2 you will notice that cholesterol is a precursor to the various sex steroid hormones, and clearly, if we have too little of it, we won't be able to produce enough of these vital chemicals. This is why overzealous reduction in cholesterol may be doing us more harm than good. Studies have found that low cholesterol levels can be associated with the development of cancer. This is because cholesterol together with other fats and proteins called lipoproteins, transport antioxidants like vitamin E and beta-carotene around your body. If you do not have enough cholesterol, your antioxidant status will be compromised as the goodies will have less means of gaining access to those free-radical nasties.

Further evidence demonstrates an association between low cholesterol and an increase in depression and even suicide. And, when we consider that cholesterol is the building block for our sex hormones, to have too little may result in diminished libidos and plummeting fertility levels.

What current wisdom tells us is that it is not cholesterol on its own that is the danger. It is only when cholesterol becomes oxidised that it becomes the villain it is so reputed to be, capable of wreaking destructive havoc on the linings of our blood vessels, culminating in the process we call atherosclerosis. Atherosclerosis is the medical term that describes the progressive blockage of our arteries, which can lead to heart attacks and strokes. How this comes about is an ideal way to move into the next section, which introduces you to the latest theories on the development of cardiovascular disease.

The New Theories

1. OXIDATION OF LDL

I'm sure most of you would have heard of LDL, the so-called 'bad cholesterol', and HDL the so-called 'good cholesterol'. LDL deposits cholesterol in your blood vessels, obviously not a good idea, whereas HDL transports cholesterol from your blood vessels to your liver where it is metabolised, and, if necessary, eliminated. If HDL levels are high and LDL levels are low you are considered to be in good shape. Well, the truth is this is only part of the story.

When your LDL becomes oxidised, this is the stage at which you will start running into trouble. How does your LDL become oxidised? In essence, this occurs when your LDL is bombarded by oxygen that has turned into free-radicals. There is just no escaping the potentially lethal effects of free-radicals. If you don't have a sufficient supply of antioxidants to neutralise their harmful effects, pretty soon you will have blood vessels that are literally choc-a-block full of oxidised LDL. This sets in motion a series of events that results in the development of deadly atheromatous plaque, and this is what blocks up your blood vessels.

Naturally, you won't realise that all this is taking place until you experience an awful chest pain and find yourself on the emergency trolley in your local hospital, surrounded by a host of young doctors pumping all sorts of quick-acting drugs into your system. You don't have to wait for a tragedy to occur before you wake up to the need to be proactive about the health of your heart. What is crucial is not merely your levels of LDL and HDL, but the extent to which your LDL is oxidised. The next question is, how would you know this?

There is a laboratory in Australia (address included at the back of this book) that measures the degree of oxidation of your cell membranes by means of a Lipid Peroxidation Test. Another very effective means of assessing the level of free-radical damage in your body is to have a Biological Terrain Assessment, which is a state-of-the-art means of evaluating a host of parameters associated with ageing. This will be discussed in the final chapter. The key issue here is your body's ability to cope with an ever-increasing free-radical load, and this hinges on your antioxidant defence system. Years of experience have led me to realise that we can't get enough of our good friends the antioxidants, so I have included a section on how you can fortify yourself with a wonderful range of new, powerful antioxidants that are particularly pertinent to the health of your heart.

Free-radical production is exacerbated by a high fat diet. If you consume a lot of fatty food that is not necessarily fresh such as deep fried foods, packaged biscuits or butter that has been stored for a long period of time, you will increase your body's burden of oxidised fats. If you recall, I mentioned earlier the connection between polyunsaturated fats and the development of inflammation. These oxidised fats have exactly the same effect, and this leads to another key process that damages your blood vessels.

2. INFLAMMATION

Inflammation is an indication that your immune system is heating up to deal with some form of threat. Recent research has identified certain types of inflammatory cells, which have fascinatingly complicated names that make them sound like something from a science fiction movie. These vascular cell adhesion molecules or VCAMS and their partners in crime—the intracellular adhesion molecules or ICAMS—respond to inflammation by recruiting cells of the immune system that greedily eat up all the fat in the area. Instead of digesting these fat cells, they become bloated with huge globules of fat, which together with oxidised LDL, form a deadly cocktail for the progression of atherosclerosis.

What cardiologists are now identifying as the primary contributing factor to the development of atherosclerosis is an event known as 'endothelial dysfunction'. The endothelium is the lining of your blood vessels, and once this area becomes damaged by oxidised LDL and inflammation, you are well on the way to harvesting serious vascular disease.

We know that free-radicals initiate the oxidation process, so now we have to uncover exactly what it is, aside from polyunsaturated fats, that triggers the inflammatory process and we're in business. Once we discover the underlying cause we can prevent the progression of events that lead to endothelial damage and the development of vascular disease.

Apart from the polyunsaturated fats, which are potent instigators of inflammation, scientists have been trying hard to uncover the other pieces in this intriguing puzzle. Although nothing is conclusive yet, certain studies suggest an association between certain micro-organisms and the development of inflammation. Helicobacter pylori, which resides in your stomach, and chlamydia pneumoniae, which is usually located in your lungs, have been linked with the elevation of a substance in your body called C-reactive protein (CRP). CRP commonly increases when inflammation is brewing, and research workers in Germany have found that when CRP goes up, so does LDL, and that atherosclerosis tends to flourish in this environment. Isn't this amazing, that a bug in the stomach could possibly lead to heart disease! This is a marvellous demonstration of the inter-relatedness of all parts of your body and how important it is to ensure maximum health in all your organs.

If you want to find out whether inflammation is fermenting somewhere in your body, have a blood test that measures the levels of CRP. This is a test that I routinely perform on my patients when I screen them for cardiovascular risk factors.

As the evidence mounts that cholesterol is merely part of a web of events that leads to coronary heart disease, it is vital that any cardiovascular surveillance includes these novel risk factors, which if detected, can be dealt with at an early stage, thereby circumventing a potential catastrophe. Healthy, middle-aged folk with normal lipid profiles (LDL and HDL levels) are at risk of developing coronary heart disease. Your CRP levels, together with an evaluation of your oxidised LDL, may provide you with information that could save your life.

If you want to prevent inflammation from taking hold in your body, in addition to dealing with its cause, you can augment your diet with anti-inflammatory nutrients. The omega-3 oils, which are found in salmon and flaxseed oil, are rich in anti-inflammatory properties that block the effects of any harmful inflammatory agents in your body. Interestingly, vitamin E, along with all its other cardiovascular benefits, protects the endothelial lining of your blood vessels from the inflammatory process that initiates atherosclerosis (3). Vitamin E should be an essential component of the nutrients you take to optimise your cardiovascular health.

3. FIBRINOGEN

Oxidation, inflammation and damage to the lining of your blood vessels are factors you have to safeguard against. Another dangerous development is the tendency of your blood to form clots. If you have plaque blocking your arteries and you form clots on top of this, you have a recipe for disaster. A heart attack is highly likely to be a consequence of this combination.

Fibrinogen forms part of the clotting system of your body, but if blood tests show that you have elevated elements of this substance, then you could be at risk of suffering a heart attack.

Some believe that raised fibrinogen levels are as significant as raised LDL in predicting the future development of heart disease. Smoking increases levels of fibrinogen, and so does a diet high in saturated fat. Women are more at risk than men in this department as they have higher levels of fibrinogen.

4. HOMOCYSTEINE

This protein has achieved major prominence as one of the new primary players in the aetiology of heart disease. It really is the cholesterol of the 21st century, but unlike cholesterol, homocysteine's effects can be remarkably deadly. It appears to exert a triple whammy in its damaging capabilities as it:

- *Promotes LDL oxidation*
- *Increases the tendency of your blood to form clots*
- *Adversely effects the endothelium which lines your blood vessels*

The tendency to develop raised homocysteine is partially diet-related and partially genetic. Its prevalence is estimated to affect between 10 and 20 per cent of the adult population. Homocysteine is formed from another protein called methionine, so if you consume a protein-enriched diet, especially one that is mostly comprised from animal protein, your levels of homocysteine may become dangerously elevated. The good news is that in the normal course of events, homocysteine is metabolised back to methionine where it makes a useful contribution to the preservation of your DNA. However, to achieve this you have to have adequate amounts of the vitamins B6,

B12 and folic acid. The bad news is that some studies have demonstrated that up to 25 per cent of the population are deficient in folic acid. In my clinical practice I have found that many of my patients are lacking effective levels of folic acid and vitamin B12. These factors could lead to a build-up of homocysteine and can accelerate the development of heart disease.

A diet rich in fruit, vegetables, nuts and seeds will boost your supply of vitamin B6 and folic acid. Chick peas, spinach, sunflower seeds, walnuts and avocados, which can form the basis of a delicious salad, are especially good sources of vitamin B6 and folic acid. Vitamin B12 is derived from organ meats, salmon, herring and egg yolk. It is also synthesised by the friendly bacteria in your gut, which is why vegetarians do not necessarily have to develop vitamin B12 deficiencies.

When you have a blood test to determine your homocysteine status, ask your doctor what your levels are. These should not exceed 14 mumol/L. If they do then you need to change your diet to one that favours a vegetarian-style of eating. In addition, I would advise you to consider taking supplementary nutrients of vitamin B6, B12 and folic acid. Certain factors will predispose you to be more at risk of raising your levels of homocysteine. These include:

- *Being an avid coffee drinker*
- *Being a member of the male sex*
- *Smoking*
- *Ageing*
- *Psychological stress*

Here is a word of caution to women. After menopause, homocysteine levels increase, and it is during this period that the fairer sex catch up to men in the development of heart disease. There is some evidence that HRT in the form of oestrogen will decrease the concentration of homocysteine in the blood (4). Recent research also demonstrates that vitamins E and C are equally protective against the effects of homocysteine, which is another justification for including these powerful antioxidants in your daily regimen (5).

5. LIPOPROTEIN (a)

Would you believe that this substance was described more than 35 years ago, and only recently has it been acknowledged as another one of the new instigators of heart disease? Lipoprotein(a) or Lp(a) is a fatty protein, and it can be viewed as a close relative of LDL. Like LDL, it deposits cholesterol on the walls of your blood vessels and it also prevents clots from dissolving.

In women, Lp(a) follows the same pattern as homocysteine. Levels become elevated after menopause (although HRT prevents this from happening). The effects of elevated Lp(a) are so devastating that raised Lp(a) levels can double the possibility of developing heart disease in middle age. We don't yet know of any dietary means of lowering Lp(a). However, if you increase your intake of vitamin C, vitamin B3 and the amino acid lysine, you will have a very effective combination of nutrients for keeping Lp(a) levels down.

6. INSULIN RESISTANCE

This is a syndrome that can have a profound impact on the ageing process. With regard to the cardiovascular system, this metabolic disorder is especially bad news. Insulin is a hormone you need to facilitate the entry of glucose into your cells where it is utilised for energy. Insulin resistance occurs when your cells become opposed to the effects of insulin, so instead of using glucose efficiently you tend to have a load of glucose racing around your body, dying to get into your cells. When your insulin starts to rise, adverse metabolic consequences tend to accumulate in your cardiovascular system. Cholesterol, LDL and fibrinogen go up, oxidant stress proliferates, while HDL goes down. Once again you have a potential calamity on your hands unless you reverse this stream of events.

This type of syndrome tends to predominate in what I call 'the sweet tooth, bread, rice and pasta brigade'. If the scales let out a groan every time you pluck up the courage to mount them, you crave chocolates and other sweet treats and find yourself tiring after a meal loaded with carbohydrates, the chances are you have insulin resistance.

A simple blood test that measures glucose and insulin before and after a carbohydrate challenge will enlighten you as to whether you are suffering from this metabolic disorder. In Chapter 9 you will receive very effective guidelines for dealing with insulin resistance.

So there you have it, *oxidised LDL, inflammation, endothelial dysfunction, homocysteine, fibrinogen, lipoprotein(a) and insulin resistance* are the new risk factors that you need to have evaluated as part of your cardiovascular program. The next time you visit your physician, insist that these parameters be measured. All of the above factors are correctable by natural means if you take action at an early stage.

The Female Sex

Heart disease was thought to reside exclusively in the masculine domain, but when we look at the statistics, women are becoming increasingly competitive in succumbing to this affliction. In fact, coronary heart disease is the leading cause of death in women. The risk of developing cardiovascular disease for women in the USA is two out of three.

To be fair, it is still important to indicate that the rates of heart disease are still higher in men than in women. The psychological profile of the average woman in the modern urban jungle is far less conducive to heart disease than men's. Women tend to share their feelings more and have extensive social supports. The type A male who exists in an aggressive, competitive and often hostile world is far more likely to drop dead from a heart attack than his female counterpart. Fascinatingly, success outside the home has not been found to be dangerous for women. Women who occupy executive, professional positions have more favourable heart disease risk factors than women who stay at home. Somehow successful women have found a way, either biologically or emotionally, to prevent the stresses of the workplace from clogging up their arteries.

From a physical perspective, women smoke less and they generally have better diets that are higher in fruits and vegetables and contain more fibre, vitamin C and folic acid—powerful protective factors. Most importantly, women have more HDL in their bloodstream.

As if the poor male does not have enough to cope with, he also has to suffer the indignity of lower HDL levels throughout his life. This is thought to be one of the major reasons why men develop atherosclerosis well before women. Naturally, hormones were thought to be primarily responsible for women's superiority in the HDL stakes, and this is where things become really interesting. When women reach menopause, HDL starts to decline and LDL goes up. You don't have to be Albert Einstein, or should I say Germaine Greer, to reach the conclusion that hormones must have something to do with these changes. Oestrogen, traditionally viewed as the most significant female hormone, has received all the praise for preserving elevated levels of HDL. When oestrogen diminishes at menopause, so does HDL. However, when we scrutinise the facts, things are not that simple.

Numerous studies have documented the benefits of taking HRT as far as heart disease is concerned. Some have even demonstrated a massive 50 per cent decrease in the incidence of heart attacks. But other variables may have contributed to these outcomes as much as HRT. The women involved in these studies who were taking HRT were also the type of women who looked after themselves. They had better diets, they exercised more, were of a higher socioeconomic status and were generally healthier than the women who were not taking HRT. Therefore, we have to question what exactly it was that resulted in such a significant reduction in heart disease. Was it the hormones, or was it those other factors?

Another very important study called the PEPI trial, which examined the relationship between different forms of HRT and heart disease, revealed that women who took oestrogen together with natural progesterone had the highest levels of HDL. This raises an interesting new perspective: maybe it's not oestrogen alone that contributes to favourable levels of HDL, and if some of the accolades are due to the effects of oestrogen, are there other means of boosting the body's natural production of oestrogen?

Companies interested in promoting natural health have not been slow to capitalise on this possibility. One such product, derived from the herb red clover, has been developed called P-081. Clinical trials indicate that this substance can boost HDL levels by 23 per cent after three months treatment. This is extremely encouraging for women who are reluctant to take oestrogen because of the possible side-effects. Nevertheless, current opinion does concede that oestrogen therapy has protective effects on the cardiovascular system. Oestrogen reduces oxidation of LDL, preserves endothelial function, decreases lipoprotein(a), homocysteine and fibrinogen levels—all considered prime initiators of heart disease in post-meno-pausal women.

What I do in my practice is to discuss all the options with my female patients, including the new form of HRT called raloxifene, which is a modified type of oestrogen that also has a favourable effect on the cardiovascular system. Then I let my patients decide what they prefer. That way they can have a positive impact on their health outcomes.

The Male Sex

Women fare better than men in the cardiovascular stakes. That's a fact. Although the margins aren't as huge as they were thought to be, they exist nevertheless. In addition to the diet and lifestyle factors already mentioned, we used to think that the other factor that made such a huge difference was hormones—women have oestrogen and that is good for the heart; while men have testosterone, which is bad. At least this has been the traditional view until now. Yes, men, I am here to tell you that you no longer have to be ashamed of those hormones that have been held responsible for pillage, war and destruction. Men were bequeathed testosterone for good reason, and for the male heart this hormone is a veritable godsend.

Testosterone was discovered to be weaving its magic as far back as 1947. Dr Maurice Lesser, considered to be one of the leading research workers of his time, demonstrated that when men suffering from long-standing angina were given testosterone their symptoms markedly improved (6). Since that time numerous studies have demonstrated the benefits of testosterone on cardiovascular health. Testosterone has a positive impact on several factors that contribute to heart disease.

These include:

• *Reducing cholesterol, blood pressure and triglycerides*
• *Decreasing fat*
• *Normalises blood glucose levels*
• *Reducing blood clotting*

In the blood there is a substance called tissue plasminogen inhibitor (t-PA), which is a very powerful dissolver of clots formed in the bloodstream. T-PA is so potent that it is currently used to treat heart-attack and stroke victims whose blood vessels are obstructed by the development of clots. A study by researchers at the University of Cincinnatti School of Medicine showed that men with higher levels of testosterone also had higher levels of t-PA. They also had lower levels of fibrinogen, which, as you now know, causes the blood to clot and lowers levels of triglycerides (11). Triglycerides are another form of fat, and having high levels of this substance can be an added risk factor for heart disease.

Testosterone increases HDL and reduces LDL. A research team headed by Dr Alan Booth at Penn State University in the USA, has recently completed a study on more than 4,300 men between the ages of 32 and 44. They found that those men who had the highest levels of testosterone had a 72 per cent lower risk of having a heart attack and a 45 per cent lower risk of having high blood pressure.

The evidence in favour of testosterone is very impressive, almost hard to ignore, and I want to reassure you that I don't have shares in any testosterone manufacturing company. Like melatonin, testosterone cannot be patented. Therefore, all this wonderful information is not so attractive to the pharmaceutical industry, and we doctors are unlikely to hear much about it unless we go searching for it. Maintaining optimal levels of testosterone is essential for cardiovascular health and I will provide you with ample means of enhancing your body's natural production of testosterone.

Before we move on, here is a word of caution to men. Oestrogen is bad for your heart. Yes, men have oestrogen in their bodies, and while this hormone is protective to the male brain, with regard to the heart, having high levels of oestrogen increases the risk of having a heart-attack. This is precisely the opposite of the female experience. How do men come to have high oestrogen levels? One of the ways is via an enzyme called aromatase, which converts testosterone to oestrogen. You might question why one of nature's substances would perform such a silly act. It's really not such a stupid intervention because we do need oestrogen for our brains as I've indicated. This is what prevents us from developing Alzheimer's disease. However, the activity of aromatase escalates with aging, obesity and when there is a deficiency of zinc and vitamin C. Doesn't nature have a wonderful sense of humour! As men age they have less chance of developing Alzheimer's, but an increased likelihood of succumbing to a heart attack. What is the moral of the story? Don't age. This may be possible if you maintain youthful levels of the anti-ageing hormones HGH, DHEA and melatonin—all of which contribute to cardiovascular health, especially DHEA. Don't get fat. This is up to you.

Have more than your fair share of zinc and vitamin C. Oysters (James Bond's favourite), beef, sunflower and pumpkin seeds are good sources of zinc, while vitamin C is found in citrus fruits, strawberries, guavas and potatoes. All this talk of food makes it an opportune time to discuss the ideal cardioprotective diet.

The Diet

It's fascinating to observe how much the perspective has shifted on the best diet for optimal cardiovascular health. In the 1960s and 1970s we thought it was a diet high in polyunsaturated fats such as margarine, and then this was discovered to be wrong. Then, in the 1980s and 1990s the experts told us to make complex carbohydrates found in bread, rice and potatoes the staple part of our diet. This is also incorrect because in some people this form of diet can promote insulin resistance, which leads to the build-up of unfavourable lipids (fats) in the body. This is definitely not good for the heart. Recent studies indicate that sugar and milk increase the incidence of heart disease (7)—information that the old dairy board would not be too happy to disseminate. Even the much denigrated egg has made a recent comeback. A study reported in the Journal of the American Medical Association tells us that having one egg per day is not bad for us after all (8). Finally, just to throw a real spanner in the works, along comes the book Eat Right 4 Your Blood Type, written by American visionary Peter D'adamo, which tells us that we need to tailor our diets to our blood type. D'adamo has even demonstrated that if you give someone with an O blood type a high protein diet with lots of meat, their HDL will actually go up and their cholesterol and triglycerides will go down. This is an outcome that we would never have anticipated given the supposed link between the consumption of animal fats and heart disease.

One man's meat is another man's poison

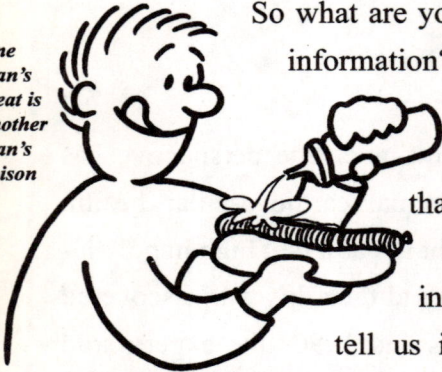

So what are you to do given all this confusing information? Is there truly an ideal diet for cardiovascular health? There are definitely certain principles that we have to observe, but before I discuss them it's important to indicate that what these findings tell us is that everybody has a unique biochemistry. One man's meat is literally another man's poison. What I do in my practice is to evaluate each patient's risk factors and then construct a program that is tailor-made to their biochemical profile. That way the best possible outcomes can be achieved given the sophisticated level of our knowledge at the present time. As a general rule I advise the following:

• Eat a diet that is rich in fruit and vegetables. These are resplendent with antioxidants that you need to keep your levels of oxidised LDL to a minimum.

• Take supplements of vitamins A, C and E. These work as a team, one replenishing the other, and they enhance the antioxidant nutrients you obtain from your diet.

• Add the B vitamins to your supplement list, especially B6, B12 and folic acid. These are necessary to deal with the harmful effects of raised homocysteine levels in your body.

Even if your blood tests for homocysteine are normal, transiently elevated levels of homocysteine, which can occur after a heavy protein meal, can be dangerous.

• Consume the good fats that are found in nuts and seeds such as walnuts, almonds and flaxseed, as well as in cold water fish such as salmon and trout. Extra-virgin olive oil and avocado will complement these nicely. Besides promoting all the favourable lipids in your body, these good fats prevent the accumulation of inflammation, which, as you remember, is toxic to your blood vessels.

• Exercise is crucial. You need to exercise at least four times a week for a minimum of 45 minutes so that you build up a sweat. Interestingly, D'adamo explains in Eat Right 4 Your Blood Type that certain blood types benefit from particular exercise programs. For example, someone with blood type A may need to do lots of yoga to calm themselves down.

In addition to the above recommendations, there are certain 'supernutrients' that can benefit your cardiovascular health immensely. Let's take a look at them.

The Proanthocyanodins

Ever since we discovered the ability of antioxidants to neutralise the effects of free-radicals, the search has been on for the ultimate antioxidant. Some scientists believe they have come close with the discovery of proanthocyanodins (OPCs), derived from such substances as red grape and maritime pine bark. These OPCs are believed to be 50 times more potent than an antioxidant such as vitamin E, and they are powerful inhibitors of LDL oxidation. This explains the so-called 'French paradox': the low incidence of heart disease among the French who consume large amounts of fatty foods together with red wine, which is rich in OPCs. This is not to encourage you to go out and drink gallons of the stuff. Certainly, one to two glasses per night would more than suffice. Post-menopausal women need to be especially conservative as exceeding this designated amount can lead to an increased risk of developing breast cancer.

COENZYME Q10

I consider this nutrient to be an essential component of everybody's cardiovascular health program. At a recent anti-ageing conference that I attended in Las Vegas, one of the presenting physicians described how the mother of his close friend became severely ill with a failing heart and pneumonia. The medical profession threw all they could at her, including drugs and the latest medical technology, and when every medical avenue failed they wrote her off. She was finally transferred to the above physician's care while on a ventilator. All she was given was Coenzyme Q10 (CoQ-10) and some other antioxidants and minerals via her nasogastric tube. After just two weeks she was discharged from hospital, nothing short of a miracle.

Your heart is made up of muscle tissue, and muscle needs energy. CoQ-10 assists the mitochondria (the powerhouse of your cell) in manufacturing ATP, which is the basic form of cellular energy. If you want to ensure that your heart muscle is pumping away as vigorously as it can, then you need to have an adequate supply of CoQ-10 on board.

CoQ-10 lowers blood pressure and is an effective inhibitor of free-radical damage. Like the OPCs, CoQ-10 reduces the oxidation of LDL quite substantially. CoQ-10 can be obtained from sources such as salmon, eggs, rice bran and peanuts, but current evidence seems to indicate that sufficient amounts cannot be obtained from dietary means alone and that supplementary CoQ-10 gives us a protective advantage.

ALPHA-LIPOIC ACID

This is another member of the 'super antioxidant family', and like CoQ-10, it facilitates the generation of ATP and prevents the oxidation of LDL. Alpha-lipoic acid has a delightfully endearing maternal role as it recycles vitamin E, which becomes a free-radical itself in its attempts to rescue LDL from the ravishes of the oxidant onslaught. Vitamin E is then able to return to the battlefields with renewed vigour and fortitude.If there is enough alpha-lipoic acid present, this renewal process can proceed indefinitely such is the strength of this nutrient.

L-CARNITINE

This is the third musketeer in the above triad of antioxidants, which includes CoQ-10 and alpha-lipoic acid. Once again, L-carnitine provides a ready source of ATP for energy. It also dilates blood vessels and increases HDL while lowering triglycerides. Arrhythmias, which are unstable heart rhythms, can be corrected by L-carnitine.

The Isoflavones

These are compounds found in substances such as soy and the herb red clover. Isoflavones enhance the resistance of LDL to oxidation, which is a good thing as it appears that LDL can't get enough support in its attempts to resist the hordes of free radicals baying for its blood. Isoflavones also have the additional bonus of increasing HDL levels. Isoflavones belong to the phyto-oestrogen family, which you will encounter repeatedly as the anti-ageing saga unfolds.

VITAMIN E

Although vitamin E appears to be playing second fiddle to a new generation of much more powerful antioxidants, it has been found to play a significant role in the prevention of heart disease. Indeed, low rates of heart disease are associated with high dietary vitamin E levels. Would you believe it if I told you that vitamin E is believed to inhibit the oxidation of LDL? Does that sound familiar? In a large experiment performed in the United Kingdom, supplements of vitamin E given in amounts exceeding those that can be obtained from dietary sources alone, significantly reduced the incidence of heart disease and heart-attacks. This was achieved in some patients who had advanced blockage of their arteries, indicating that if oxidation of LDL is the culprit this can be reversed by high-dose antioxidants.

MAGNESIUM

This is a mineral that is vital for cardiovascular health, and it's a nutrient that most of us don't get enough of in our diets. This is because the foods that are highest in magnesium such as vegetables (especially legumes and dark green vegetables), whole-grains and nuts, are not major constituents of our daily diets. Magnesium deficiency is associated with all the manifestations of heart disease, including irregular heart beat, increasing atherosclerosis, raised blood pressure and heart attack. Magnesium supplementation has been shown to lower blood pressure and prevent the development of atherosclerosis by reducing total cholesterol and raising HDL.

This chapter would not be complete without a mention of two other important factors—chelation therapy and the importance of an open heart.

CHELATION THERAPY

A clinic has recently opened in Sydney, offering the latest in high-tech scanning for evaluating the extent to which atherosclerosis is present in coronary arteries. A correlation has been made between the amount of calcification and the degree to which coronary arteries are obstructed. Enter chelation therapy. Chelation therapy is a process whereby a substance called Ethylene Diamine Tetra Acetic acid (EDTA) is administered, which removes calcium and the other heavy metals such as lead, aluminium and iron, all of which may initiate the free-radical process that results in the oxidation of LDL. This is a very effective means of preventing the accumulation of the atherosclerotic material that gums up your blood vessels. Certainly it's a far less painful procedure than having coronary artery by-pass surgery.

Opening Your Heart

Although I've relegated this segment to the final item on optimising cardiovascular health, this is not to diminish its importance. Having an open heart in the emotional sense is vital to everybody's health. Experiments have demonstrated that ongoing emotional deprivation and the absence of normal social contacts leads to coronary artery blockages regardless of the levels of oxidised LDL. Further studies have shown that patients make quicker recoveries after a heart attack if they are encouraged to have a daily association with a pet. We all know how open-hearted pets such as cats and dogs can be. If you haven't yet discovered the partner of your dreams, then man's best friend may be the next best option.

Key Points To Remember

The new risk factors for heart disease include:
• Oxidised LDL
• Inflammation
• Fibrinogen
• Homocysteine
• Lipoprotein(a)
• Insulin resistance

Have these assessed as a matter of priority!

The nutrients that ensure optimal cardiovascular health include:

- Vitamins A, C, E, B6, B12 and folic acid
- Proanthocyanodins found in red grape and maritime pine bark extract
- Coenzyme Q-10
- Alpha-lipoic acid
- L-carnitine
- Magnesium

CHAPTER 5

Boosting Brain Power

Boosting
Brain Power

*I*MAGINE THIS: TOM AND SARAH ARE INVITED TO A PARTY. TOM IS a 43-year-old lawyer—bright, witty and successful. Sarah is a 38-year-old accounts executive in a prominent company in the city. When he arrives at the party, Tom is introduced to a number of the guests. Finally he meets Sarah and he listens attentively to a detailed account of a business transaction that she was recently involved in, even though to the average listener this may appear somewhat boring. He then entertains her with a blow-by-blow description of a recent golfing weekend that he enjoyed with friends. At the end of the conversation she gives him her work number, which he commits to memory. A week later he phones her and they are both able to share amusing recollections of interactions they had with various guests at the party, remembering each guest by name. They can also both recall specifics of their conversation, which serves to brighten the connection they are forging with each other.

Consider this: same party different players. George is a 41-year-old senior partner at one of the leading accounting practices in the city. He is a renowned culinary expert and a good golfer. Mary is a 39-year-old physician who has recently established a solo practice in a fashionable eastern suburb. When they are ultimately introduced to each other, they have both met so many people that they can't remember who is Arthur and who is Martha. At the end of their conversation, Mary gives George her phone number, which he writes down on a piece of paper. Three days later when he decides that this is the time to rekindle the flames that he thought were ignited, he attempts to retrieve the piece of paper upon which he had inscribed her phone number. He can't remember where he put the piece of paper, nor can he recall the name of the gentleman who introduced the two of them. When he finally secures her number by a very circuitous route, she struggles to remember who he is or any of the details of the conversation they had only three nights previously.

Does the second scenario seem more familiar to you? The moral of the story? Mary and George were so drunk that they couldn't remember a thing. No, that's not it. Lawyers and accounts executives have better memories than accountants and physicians. Wrong again. Tom and Sarah were able to retrieve information in such impressive detail because they have trained their minds to operate on such a level. They have realised how important it is to have a good memory and they have actively gone about cultivating mind power in this area. They are not necessarily gifted, nor is it likely that they were born with superior capabilities. They have simply committed themselves to developing the skills needed to retrieve large amounts of information.

Think about the top 100 tennis players in the world. What is it that separates them? Is it their skills? Are the top 10 players so much more gifted or talented than the players who occupy positions 90 to 100? Not necessarily. On his day the 95th player could beat the world number one if he simply did one thing. Some of you will know what I am getting at. Yes, if that player put his mind to it, then there is every possibility that he could give the number one player in the world a real run for his money. The power of the mind is probably the key factor that separates these athletes, all of whom are at the peak of their chosen careers. Pat Rafter has acknowledged that one of the practices that helped him to win the American Open was the ability he developed to meditate during the change-overs. This allowed him to calm his mind right down so that he was refreshed and ready for the next game.

The great achievers of our time, be they sports people, actors, politicians or academics, have reached the pinnacle of their profession mostly because they have absolutely and totally committed to excellence in their field and they have utilised every atom of their mind to succeed. Genes, talents and innate gifts have their place, but as these people will tell you it is 10 percent inspiration and 90 percent perspiration. Developing and training the mind to its full potential is what separates these so-called supermen from us mere mortals. They have set themselves goals and they have remained singularly focused in the fulfilment of their mission. Perhaps you could scale the heights of Everest if you set your mind to it.

You see, in some ways your brain is similar to your biceps. This doesn't mean that it has limited neuronal connections. On the contrary. What I am getting at is that like your muscles, your brain can be developed almost infinitely. I often gaze in awe and admiration at the magnificent physiques of some of the more regular attendees at the local gym. Countless hours are spent painstakingly cultivating the perfect body. Think how evolved we would be if similar loving attention was devoted to perfecting our brain muscles. When you marvel at the sophistication of today's computers, take the time to bask in the achievements of the human brain. The computer didn't design itself. It was someone like you or me who developed this wondrous machine. The world chess champion is able to consistently beat the smartest computer around. Now, not all of us may be as clever as he is, but this feat clearly indicates that the human mind is capable of superhuman achievements.

Too often I hear patients lamenting that their mental and physical faculties are deteriorating. Last year I commenced an early-morning walking club to initiate a regular exercise routine with my patients while having some fun at the same time. Fun, by the way, should be part of everybody's anti-ageing program and a substantial part of your average day. I try to have as much fun as I can with my patients, given that illness is a pretty serious affair. On one particular day I overheard one of the participants remarking—and this was an exceptionally fit young man in his early 40s—that he no longer intended to do any jogging as he was getting old and this type of exercise was bad for his bones. Sadly, I reflected on the negative impact that this kind of message must be sending to his body.

Just as you can think your body into old age, so you can age your brain prematurely. Patients who express their concern about rapidly diminishing memories often report this kind of circumstance with reluctant resignation, as if their brains were sliding inexorably into inevitable decline. Although there is undoubtedly some aspects of mental functioning that do drop off with age, the brain is a remarkably plastic organ that can develop new nerve connections and strengthen existing communication pathways at virtually any age. This is what Dr Robert Goldman, Director of the American Academy of Anti-Ageing Medicine, informs us in his book entitled Brain Fitness.(1). The old adage 'use it or you lose it' as Dr Goldman indicates, is especially applicable in this area. However, even if you lose it, certain faculties can be regained. In one truly astonishing experiment, a group of researchers took a select number of 70-year-olds whose ability to solve problems and perform spatial orientation tasks, like read maps, had deteriorated. The researchers gave the group only five hours of training in learning spatial relationships and problem-solving exercises. Much to their surprise and delight 40 per cent of the participants regained the mental skills that they had lost, and what was even more staggering was that they retained what they had learned a full seven years later.

The same research team then went on to establish what it was amongst older people that preserved their mental functions and kept their minds alive and sharp. They found that these folk shared certain qualities:

• They regularly did a variety of activities including reading, travelling and joining professional organisations.

• They were married or involved with a bright partner.

• Some, although not all, retained employment or were professionally active.

• They were able to grasp new concepts and were open to change.

• They generally had a sunny outlook on life.

I constantly marvel at the mental disposition of my mother. It was not so long ago that she mastered Windows-95 and was the director of a large library that had a substantial number of staff. She is currently helping me find my way around the computer, which requires a certain amount of patience and a lot of humour.

The Mini Mental Test

To get a sense of how well your grey matter is firing and whether your neuronal connections are being preserved, complete the following mini-mental assessment. What you need to do is rate each of the following symptoms:

Scale: 0 = never, 1 = occasionally, 2 = frequently

• Poor memory
• Inability to concentrate
• Learning disabilities
• Difficulty in making decisions
• Confusion
• Problems with comprehension

Scores:

0:      Congratulations, perhaps you could share your secrets with us.

1–5:   You are not in immediate danger of mental decline although you should not take your mind for granted.

6-9:   You need to pay a lot of attention to the advice in this chapter and get a friend to quiz you on the main points.

10-12: Fast forward to the section on 'supernutrients' to boost brain power. Take these until you have cleared away the cobwebs and then continue reading.

Exercising The Mind

When it comes to boosting brain power, the key point you need to understand is that you have to actively engage in intellectual pursuits that challenge your mind.

• Learn how to speed read. This involves scanning new material by reading the first and the last sentence in each paragraph to get the gist of what is being stated. Try it now with this chapter and then return to read the whole segment and compare the difference in your level of retention and comprehension of the main points.

• Learn new words from the dictionary each week and commit these to memory. When you come across words you don't understand in a piece that you are reading, look these up and memorise them. Quiz yourself to see how many words you remember. Try these new words out in conversation with friends. Not only will this impress them, but they will be acquiring a new repertoire as well.

• Learn a new language. Now there's a challenge. What's even more fun is learning a new musical instrument. That way you are integrating both sides of your brain and you will be establishing new neuronal connections, which is the key to building stronger mind power.

• Resist using your calculator until you have done the necessary calculations in your head, and then check your adding skills so that you don't erode your valuable lunch break correcting your errors.

• Use your other hand for writing as often as you can. No matter how embarrassing this looks, your brain will appreciate the effort.

• Play mental games with yourself. What I like to do is focus on the number plate of a motorcar, find the highest number, and then combine the other numbers in various permutations so that they add up to this number. When I was younger I used to play a card game that is very similar to this exercise.

• Think of five new ways to make a fortune and put them into practice. If any of them succeed, inform the author of this book before you tell your friends.

I love to watch children play. The way they incorporate their imaginations is truly astounding. You can utilise the above exercises in the same fashion. Enjoy being creative and reap the benefits of this new expansiveness.

Memory

Of all the mental functions that decline with age, a diminishing memory is surely the most alarming and the most debilitating. As the following graphs illustrate, this decline is steady and persistent.

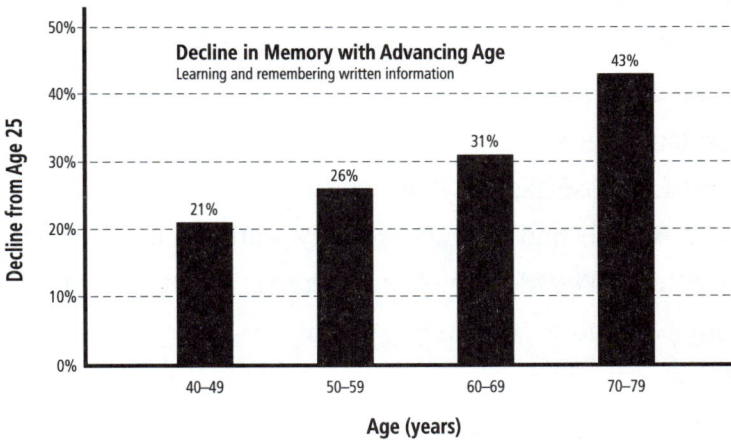

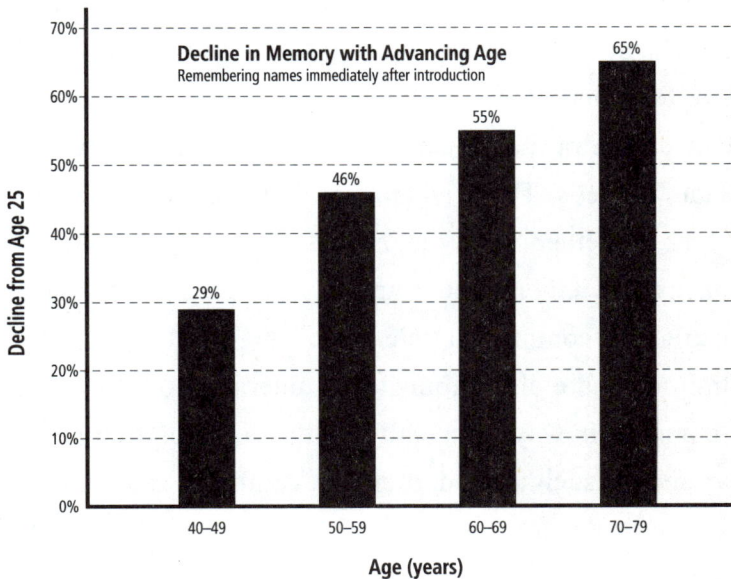

Decline in Memory with Advancing Age
Learning and remembering written information

Age (years)	Decline from Age 25
40–49	21%
50–59	26%
60–69	31%
70–79	43%

Decline in Memory with Advancing Age
Remembering names immediately after introduction

Age (years)	Decline from Age 25
40–49	29%
50–59	46%
60–69	55%
70–79	65%

We seem to have most trouble with the recall of short-term events as well as the retrieval of information stored in long-term memory banks. Most of you are familiar with the embarrassment of forgetting the names of people to whom you were recently introduced, or the frustration of trying to retrieve information you have learned at university, only to find your memory fails you time and time again. I think it is fair to say that the majority would consider this a fact of life and something you can do very little about. But there is a lot you can do to resuscitate your ailing memory. In order to do this you have to understand those factors that lead us to forget so readily. As Thomas Crook and Brenda Adderly indicate in a masterful work entitled The Memory Cure, there are a number of reasons for the weakening of memory with age.

1. THE AGEING OF OUR BRAIN CELLS

Unlike other cells, our brain cells are exquisitely sensitive to the absence of essential nutrients. Deprive a brain cell of oxygen for a matter of minutes and it will die. This is why you have to take extra special care to provide your brain with all the nutrients it needs. The B vitamins, which include B1, B3, B6 and B12, together with the minerals zinc, magnesium and boron, are all vital brain nutrients. My experience indicates that these are very common deficiencies.

Brain cells are also exquisitely vulnerable to all the toxins that come their way, especially in the form of free-radicals. Heavy metals such as lead, mercury, cadmium and aluminium contribute to the free-radical load that is so harmful to brain tissue. Much has been spoken of aluminium's role as a causative agent for Alzheimer's disease, and although this has never been proven, there are studies to show that Alzheimer's patients are more likely to have lived in areas where the concentration of aluminium in the water supply is high (3). These and other research findings have been enough to scare most people about the dangers of aluminium. I don't know anybody these days who would consider using aluminium cookware. If you are concerned about the build-up of aluminium or any other heavy metals, have a hair mineral analysis that will give you a complete breakdown of the heavy metal load in your body.

Smoking and excessive alcohol consumption (more than two glasses of red wine per night) are extremely harmful to brain tissue, directly by the damage they cause and by the proliferation of free-radicals they induce. Excess homocysteine is as damaging to the brain as it is to the heart. Some research even suggests that this substance may be linked to Alzheimer's disease. Inflammation that eats away at your blood vessels has an equally pernicious effect on your brain. So you can see that the very principles that apply to your cardiovascular health are very pertinent to the health of your brain, only your brain needs that much more tender loving care.

For your brain to function effectively, messages have to be relayed from one nerve cell to the next and this is achieved by means of special chemicals

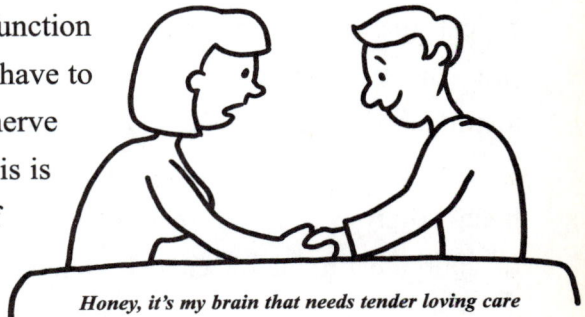

Honey, it's my brain that needs tender loving care

called neurotransmitters. Memory, comprehension, learning, mood states and all the other higher mental processes are dependant on adequate supplies of these essential brain chemicals. Acetylcholine is the neurotransmitter responsible for memory, concentration and learning; dopamine is the feel-good neurotransmitter that you turn on with sensual pleasures; and serotonin prevents you from feeling down in the dumps. Ageing results in a diminished supply of neurotransmitters, probably due to poor diets and digestive systems that don't absorb all the nutrients necessary to make up these substances. In The Memory Cure, Crook has even been so bold as to claim that the difference between Alzheimer's and the decline in memory with age is only one of degree. To substantiate this he says that the neurotransmitter supply drops off in both instances, although in Alzheimer's disease this reduction is more marked. Before all of you with memory problems hit the panic button, these are only views expressed by Crook. Alzheimer's is a little more than a mere reduction in neuro-transmitters as you will shortly discover.

Another critical component of normal brain function is cell membranes. For the neurotransmitters to relay their chemical messages they have to be recognised, received and relayed by cell membranes that surround your cells. Cell membranes prevent cells from becoming over-excited by incoming stimulation and they generally repel any input that is toxic to your cells, pretty much like your good old fairy godmother. By being so protective, cell membranes allow your mitochondria to continue producing energy, unhindered. Cell membranes are also subject to age related decline. Because they are mostly made up of fats that can go rancid very easily, cell membranes are prone to disaster if free-radicals take hold. In the 'supernutrient' section, you will get a special preview of a nutrient that promises to revolutionise brain health by safeguarding the wellbeing of your cell membranes.

2. POOR NUTRITION AND LACK OF EXERCISE

We are a culture largely guilty of the malnutrition of excess. Instead of eating a good supply of foods that provide healthy nutrients for our brain cells, we tend to load up on empty calories that mostly consist of fats. These may taste nice, but their nutrient value is limited. If they were the good fats found in nuts, seeds and fish this would be beneficial, but instead they are the fats found in animal products that can increase the free-radical load as well as inflammation. Our poor brain cells are the first to pay the price for this kind of lifestyle. Eating too much also adds to the free-radical burden, and if this is compounded by a lifestyle that is devoid of exercise, then it's no wonder that memories diminish and brains become sluggish and slow.

3. THE TELEVISION CULTURE

Dr Bob Goldman tells us that in order to memorise a piece of information we have to focus on it, organise it and process it. Repetition helps to send information to the long-term memory storage bank so that it can be retrieved at a later stage. This kind of mental activity demands that we challenge our minds to be mentally active. Spending long hours in front of the television will not provide your mind with the kind of endeavour it needs to keep those memory cells ticking over. Once you stop challenging yourself to learn and remember new material, your brain cells will start to atrophy or shrink, which will make it even harder for you the next time around, and on you will go in an endless downward spiral.

4. STRESS

This is probably the single most destructive chemical force in people's lives. Stress that is ongoing, unremitting and unresolved leads to a steady stream of the hormone cortisol, which can cause tissue damage, confusion and even dementia. Persistently elevated levels of cortisol have an inhibitory effect on learning and memory. This effect is most strikingly demonstrated on that part of the brain primarily responsible for memory, namely the hippocampus. The brain is dependent on glucose for energy, and cortisol prevents glucose from being transported into the cells of the hippocampus. Once glucose becomes unavailable, the mitochondria are unable to produce enough energy to sustain your cells, and mental functions become severely compromised. Studies have confirmed that individuals who have a continuously elevated production of cortisol have signif- icant memory and learning deficits, which reflect endangered hippocampal function. Along with all the other possible causes, prolonged production of high levels of cortisol is now considered one of the biggest risk factors for Alzheimer's disease, which leads us to the fifth major cause of memory loss.

5. ALZHEIMER'S DISEASE

Of all the dreaded diseases of ageing this is probably the one that lurks in the upper recesses of most people's consciousness. When people discover that their memory isn't what it used to be often their first thought is: "Am I getting Alzheimer's?" In the majority of cases this fear is misplaced. As I've indicated, we all go through some form of memory decline. Unless this is associated with confusion, changes in personality and the inability to remember familiar tasks like operating a washing machine, then it is not likely you have Alzheimer's disease.

Although there are lots of possibilities, we still have a lot to discover about the cause of Alzheimer's disease. We know there is a gene called apoE4 that increases the likelihood of contracting Alzheimer's, but it does not make the outcome an absolute certainty. Women are more at risk of contracting Alzheimer's than men, partially because of the protective effects of oestrogen. "How does this work," I hear you ask? "Isn't oestrogen the female hormone?" It sure is, but after menopause oestrogen production declines, whereas men have an enzyme called aromatase that converts the male hormone testosterone into oestrogen. Therefore, men have enough oestrogen to protect their brain cells. Kind of a cruel joke, don't you think?

The memory loss of Alzheimer's disease is typified by the inability to remember how to perform familiar activities. Also, you may be able to remember what happened years ago but not who you had tea with this morning. There is no single definitive test for Alzheimer's, which is why it's so difficult to reassure people they don't have the disease. Usually it takes eight to 10 years to succumb to this devastating affliction, which typically goes through three stages starting with confusion and memory loss. This is followed by wandering and pacing as well as difficulty with carrying out daily activities. Finally the disease culminates in the loss of control of bodily functions and total dependence on the assistance of others.

Free-radicals, homocysteine, inflammation, elevated cortisol levels, aluminium and a decline in the neurotransmitter acetylcholine, which is responsible for learning and memory, have all been nominated as possible causes, but we don't yet have a complete handle on this mystifying illness. However, astounding new research may just have an explanation for the ravages that this disease progressively exerts on the body. As you now know, for brain cells to maintain effective functioning, cell membranes have to preserve their stability. When over-exposed to neurotoxins, chemicals, free-radicals and an abundance of heavy metals such as mercury and lead, cell membranes become overexcited. A series of chemical events are then set in motion that your cell membranes are unable to repel. Free-radicals then multiply and your cells are left defenceless at the hands of these metabolic invaders. The mitochondria are the most vulnerable components of your cells and they undergo decimation on a grand scale. With no energy, brain cells die and the culmination of this process is the disease we know as Alzheimer's disease. This is not yet proven scientific fact, but evidence is mounting to support this hypothesis. If it turns out to be correct, it will offer all of us tremendous hope. It will mean that Alzheimer's disease can be prevented if we take the necessary precautions.

If you become proactive, not only will you supercharge your memory faculties but you will fortify yourself against the dreaded degenerative diseases of ageing. Let's take a look at how you can achieve the same recall abilities as our protagonists at the beginning of this chapter. Remember them?

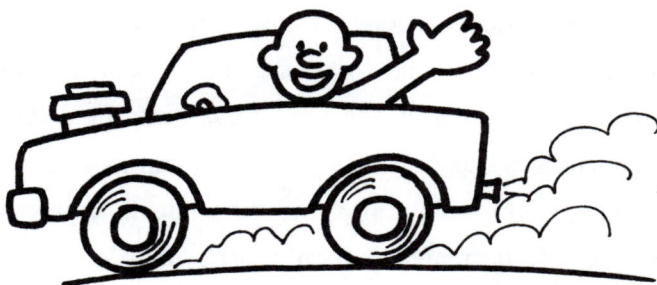

Turbocharging Your Memory

1. DIET AND NUTRITION

To protect your brain cells and boost your memory you have to consume an antioxidant-rich diet similar to the one that enhances cardiovascular health. Lots of fruit, vegetables, nuts, seeds and fish will once again provide you with the necessary platform for optimal mind power. Taking supplements of the vitamins A, C and E will augment your antioxidant defences. Studies indicate that antioxidant deficiencies may accelerate cognitive decline. In a recent study, vitamin E was shown to delay the progression of Alzheimer's disease quite substantially (4). It is also believed to ward off the memory problems associated with ageing. Together with vitamin C, vitamin E may protect against cognitive impairment (5).

Many of the B vitamins—B1, B3, B5, B6 and B12—enhance cognitive activity and memory by contributing to the synthesis of key neurotransmitters such as acetylcholine, dopamine and serotonin. The production of adequate levels of acetylcholine is critical to memory. Having optimal levels of vitamin B1 will prevent confusion, forgetfulness and depression. Vitamin B3 improves energy production and is necessary for a number of biochemical reactions that occur in the body. Vitamin B5 is known as the anti-stress vitamin. Vitamin B6 activates thinking and memory skills. Vitamin B12 prevents nerve damage by maintaining the fatty sheath that surrounds nerves. If left untreated, vitamin B12 deficiency can lead to severe brain and nerve impairment. By consuming green vegetables, brown rice, tofu, nuts, sunflower seeds and eggs, you should be getting a good supply of the B vitamins.

Certain minerals are considered to be important for memory. Boron, found in apples, pears and beans, improves alertness and learning. Zinc is another memory mineral, a deficiency of which has been linked to confusion and dementia in the elderly. Zinc is obtained by consuming beef, oysters, ginger, herring, beans and peas. Magnesium is good for your circulation and prevents calcification from eroding your neurones (brain cells). Almonds, cashews, soybeans, seafood and blackstrap molasses provide magnesium in abundance. The nutritional supplement lecithin, derived from soybean oil, is a good source of choline. Choline is the building block for acetylcholine, the neurotransmitter primarily responsible for comprehension, learning and memory.

2. EXERCISE

Exercise floods your brain with oxygen and other nutrients that keep your memory pathways well oiled. There are even studies that prove those who exercise regularly improve their memory skills and general level of mental performance far more than those who lead sedentary lives. One excellent tip that I've picked up from mind power expert Dr Bob Goldman is to intersperse short bursts of exercise with long periods of work. I have found this to be a wonderful means of recharging my batteries.

3. HORMONES FOR SMARTS

A lot of experimental evidence is now pointing to the fact that oestrogen significantly improves learning and memory. This has regenerated interest in hormone replacement therapy because these studies substantiate oestrogen's considerable benefits in upgrading memory and a host of other mental functions. Oestrogen stimulates the production of a substance called Nerve Growth Factor, which protects the brain cells vital for memory. The production of acetylcholine receives a major boost from the presence of oestrogen. This probably contributes to women on HRT showing a greater ability to remember telephone numbers and directions. The most impressive statistic of all is provided by a 16-year-long study at Johns Hopkins Bayview Medical Centre in the US, which shows that women on HRT have a dramatic 50 per cent reduction in Alzheimer's disease. Furthermore, women who do not take HRT in the form of oestrogen are 2.3 times more likely to have Alzheimer's (6).

The anti-ageing hormones DHEA and HGH (human growth hormone) also play a part in revitalising memory. By counteracting the effect of the stress hormone cortisol, DHEA makes it easier for the hippocampus, which is responsible for memory, to do its thing. Although we still have a lot to learn with respect to HGH and its effect on the brain, it too seems to enhance memory.

4. AEROBICS FOR THE MIND

If you want to take full advantage of a memory boosting program, not only do you have to exercise and eat well, but you have to put your memory cells through a training schedule similar to the workout you would regularly have at the gym. How good is your memory? Take the following test, which has been modified from Dr Goldman's work, to get an idea of how you are performing relative to your age. Read through the following list once, turn it over, and then write down how many items you remember.

• tomato	• lettuce	• garlic	• orange
• water	• lemon	• chocolate	• red wine
• rice	• watermelon	• horseradish	• turnip
• tangerine	• apple	• potato	• butternut
• zucchini	• coconut		

Scoring:	*Age*	*Normal*
	18 to 39	10 items
	40 to 59	9 items
	60 to 69	8 items
	70 and above	7 items

Do you have the memory of a much older person? Realise that you are probably not alone. Most of us are guilty of letting our memory powers wane. A good place to start is to find out how you remember. About 65 percent of us are visual learners. We remember best if we see written information or we form visual images of what we want to remember. Writing down lists of the activities you have to do might help to jog your memory. What I find useful is writing notes when I attend a lecture based on my own summation of the main points, rather than copying them from the visual material. I then revise what I have written. This way I have focused on the material, repeated it, and formed a mental picture of what I've recently learned.

Fifteen per cent of us are kinesthetic learners. This means that we remember best by connecting the situation with movement. Athletes do this by imitating and memorising elaborate movements to perfect their sporting achievements. The other 20 per cent of us are auditory learners. Auditory repetition helps us to transpose items from the short-term to the long-term memory bank. The next time you want to remember something, try saying it out loud and note whether this helps you. Give yourself a day's break and then return to the above list and try out the different memory styles (obviously not directly after each other). You can use all of these memory techniques to improve your recall abilities.

A fun way to improve your memory is to use offbeat visual images. I recently met a gentleman whose last name corresponded to the name of a well-known motor vehicle.

What I did was imagine his face on the front of the vehicle and I had no trouble remembering his name. Naturally, not all your visual images have to be as bizarre and as elaborate as this, but if you can make them slightly idiosyncratic, shall we say, then your memory will be better for it. Adding vivid colour will also help to consolidate the image in your memory. Associations and alliterations will make it easier for you to remember names. For example: Shawn who is short and says too much.

5. DEALING WITH STRESS

One of the biggest hurdles we all have to overcome is dealing effectively with stress. This phenomenon is unavoidable in everyday living. Coping with and processing stress so that its effects are energising rather than debilitating is one of the major accomplishments of any anti-ageing program. Remember, persistent stress and chronically elevated cortisol is the number one enemy of your memory.

The easiest and most effective way I know for dealing with stress is to learn the age-old practice of transcendental meditation. This will align your stress hormones by elevating your levels of DHEA, calming you down and making you feel more relaxed. Transcendental meditation is a technique for relaxing the mind by bringing about a state of mental stillness and quiet. This method of meditation also reduces anxiety and is very easy to learn. All you need is a comfortable position, a quiet environment and a non-engaging mind. Try this for yourself now.

Find a quiet space and sit in a relaxed comfortable position. Choose a word or phrase that you can repeat in your mind, and once you have become relaxed by slowing down your breathing, start to say this word quietly and repeatedly. Allow whatever thoughts come into your mind to be there, then let them go and return to your word. Continue this for 10 to 20 minutes, then slowly return your awareness to your body, open your eyes and have a stretch. Repeat this procedure every day and you will be modulating your cortisol levels so that they do not harm your brain in any way. In addition to this very simple technique, there is a nutrient available that can reduce stress levels while boosting memory and numerous other mental functions. Now let's turn to the memory 'supernutrients'. You've already heard about the heart supernutrients, some of which are the brain supernutrients as well. They are that versatile.

Memory and Mind Power Supernutrients

PHOSPHATIDYLSERINE

Phosphatidylserine (PS), one of the new kids on the block, is arguably the cream of the brain supernutrients. Derived from soy lecithin, it has an impressive array of talents:

• It reduces the effects of stress by suppressing the hormones that bring about cortisol release.

• It protects and safeguards cell membranes, thereby preventing premature brain ageing.

• It is responsible for nerve growth regulation and reverses the decline of Nerve Growth Factor in the hippocampus— the memory centre.

• It has antioxidant properties and is able to protect cells against the harmful attack of free-radicals.

• It enhances acetylcholine and dopamine release, which boosts your memory and makes you feel good. This probably has the most profound impact on preventing any form of cognitive decline.

• It can renew memory by 14 years.

Studies show that PS improves short-term memory, mental sharpness, ability to maintain concentration and long-term recall. In one landmark trial, Dr Crook of The Memory Cure fame demonstrated the ability of PS to rejuvenate memory by a staggering 14 years. As Figure 7 indicates, those who took

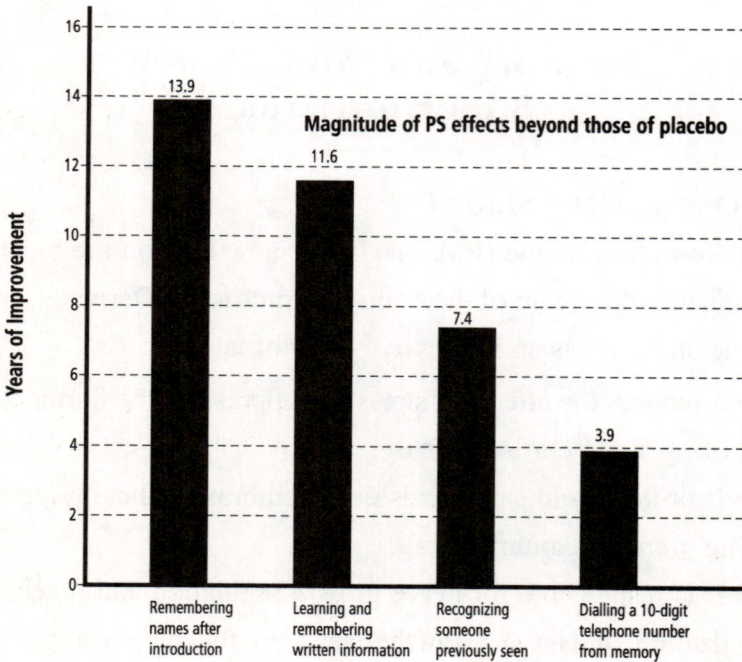

Magnitude of PS effects beyond those of placebo

Figure 7.

PS for a mere 12 weeks experienced an age-related reversal of nearly 14 years in their ability to learn and remember names after introduction. Significant improvements were also achieved with learning and concentration (7). There isn't another drug or nutrient that comes as close to achieving this kind of astronomical regeneration of mental powers.

PS is able to alleviate depression by elevating mood. It can also benefit Alzheimer's sufferers at every stage of the disease; even those who are severely compromised experience improvement after commencing PS. Athletes use PS to enhance their performance as it antagonises the effects of cortisol, which is known to cause muscle breakdown. PS has also been shown to stimulate spikes of growth hormone release, which is another huge bonus of this amazing nutrient. Although PS is far more abundant in the brain than in any other organ, it is also known to be involved in the maintenance of bones, testicular function and the elimination of ageing red cells from the blood.

GINKGO BILOBA

Ginkgo biloba is another extremely versatile brain nutrient that contributes to the prolongation of mental acuity. Like PS, ginkgo has the distinctive ability to influence mental function and behaviour. Since 1975 there have been numerous studies that document ginkgo's profound impact on intellectual function. In Germany, ginkgo has been prescribed by countless practitioners to treat memory loss.

Ginkgo has the following capabilities:

• It is a potent antioxidant that protects red blood cells from free-radical damage, thereby ensuring the safe passage of oxygen to your brain cells.

• It improves the brain's ability to utilise glucose.

• It has anti-stress and anxiety relieving actions.

A number of studies have confirmed ginkgo's efficacy in treating patients with Alzheimer's dementia and those suffering from the effects of stroke. Short-term memory, intelligence, mood and emotional stability are all noted to be considerably improved. Ginkgo is the ideal medicine for disorders relating to restricted blood flow to the brain, as well as for the customary deficits of ageing such as memory decline and poor concentration.

Both PS and ginkgo biloba can be incorporated into your strategy to preserve higher mental capacities while significantly boosting your mental powers.

ALPHA-LIPOIC ACID

This nutrient is a potent antioxidant that plays a very important role in protecting cell membranes and shielding the mitochondria from any of the dangerous effects of free-radicals. Alpha-lipoic acid also chelates or binds to heavy metals, thereby rendering them harmless.

ACETYL-L-CARNITINE

This is another of the crucial nutrients needed for the fight against premature brain ageing. Acetyl-l-carnitine (ALC) is L-carnitine with an acetyl group added, which allows ALC to enter your brain.

ALC does the following:

• It increases the production of acetylcholine and dopamine, which boosts learning, memory and emotional stability.

• It is a vital brain antioxidant that prevents the accumulation of lipofuscin granules in the hippocampus. Having lipofuscin building up in the hippocampus is like having rancidity progressively erode your mental faculties and rot your brain.

• Studies show that supplementation with ALC may impede the progression of Alzheimer's disease, and in some cases can achieve considerable improvements.

Because the neurotransmitters are so centrally important in the preservation and enhancement of normal mental functioning, if you find that you are having lapses in memory and your higher mental powers are deteriorating, then it would be wise to undertake the appropriate tests that will inform you whether you have adequate levels of acetylcholine and dopamine.

So what have you learned? By having the right diet and supplementary nutrient program, and regularly doing a brain workout, which can be just as much fun as any form of exercise, you can optimise your brain power. Then you will be able to lock horns with any computer, and you may just remember the names of guests at parties.

Key Points To Remember

Optimal brain power depends on:
• An antioxidant rich diet
• Regular mental and memory aerobics
• Daily intake of supplementary vitamins, minerals and supernutrients

The enemies of your brain are:
- Heavy metal toxins
- Free-radicals
- Homocysteine
- Excessive consumption of animal fats
- Unresolved stress

Brain Boosters include:
- Meditation
- Phosphatidylserine
- Ginkgo biloba
- Alpha-lipoic acid
- Acetyl-l-carnitine

Preventing Cancer

Preventing Cancer

ONE OF THE MOST DAUNTING ORDEALS THAT I HAVE TO FACE IS telling someone they have cancer. Imagine yourself sitting in a doctor's office waiting for the news of your test with agonising anticipation and your worst fears are confirmed. Very little could be more traumatic than receiving this type of information, and for some it can be the equivalent of a death sentence. Even though today's treatments, either conventional or alternative, are becoming more sophisticated, all too often this devastating illness leads to the experience of endless suffering, both physical and emotional. I've had the misfortune of witnessing some dreadful demises, and in many ways the end may have been a welcome relief. I'll never understand why nature would want to toy with us in such a merciless fashion. Nevertheless, cancer and all its harrowing consequences is a fact of life.

The truth is none of us need ever get this dreaded disease. Cancer is 100 per cent preventable. I'm here to tell you that each and every one of you can absolutely and totally, for your whole lives, avoid this awful illness. The trick is knowing how. I'm going to let you in on a little secret—it's easy if you make the right choices. The essence of this exercise is committing yourself to prudent health practices. Even if the genetic dice is loaded against you, you can still impact on your constitution in a way that will avert any potential disaster. However, you have to make a concerted effort.

It is not wise to leave things to chance as current trends in the USA indicate that 42 per cent of all males and 39 per cent of all females are expected to develop cancer at some stage in their lives. The incidence of breast and prostate cancer is 11 per cent and 12 per cent respectively, and these figures appear to be increasing. What is even more astounding is that 75 to 80 per cent of cancers are caused by factors associated with poor lifestyle habits such as smoking, excessive alcohol consumption and imperfect diets. Bad nutrition is considered to occupy the lion's share of this statistic. You may not have total control over an unfavourable environment but you can decide what you put in your mouth. By simply adopting a cancer-preventing diet you can radically alter the course of your life. It's therefore important to understand how cancers develop so that you can take the necessary precautions.

The Development and Prevention of Cancer

Most cancers take a long, long time to grow and become clinically evident. In some cases it may take up to three decades before anything suspicious starts to happen. At each and every stage in this process, nutritional intervention can change the outcome. Cancer is the culmination of years of pathological reactions and it is never too soon to intervene. Diets high in animal fats, sugars and excessive calories are considered to be cancer-promoting as they lead to the accumulation of free-radicals. Conversely, diets high in fruit and vegetables contain antioxidants aplenty and are cancer protective.

In the beginning, harmful agents from the environment such as toxic chemicals, UV radiation and certain viruses will be acted upon by oxygen to generate what is called reactive oxygen species, which is another term for free-radicals. These substances are highly dangerous and if they are allowed free reign they will attack the DNA of your cells. The DNA is the most fundamental and vital component of your cellular structure as it contains the genetic blueprint that governs the replication of your cells. If this basic genetic code is impaired and your DNA starts to mutate or alter, then abnormal cells may start to replicate, which can become cancer cells. There are two essential questions that you need to be asking right now. The first is, how can you prevent this process from taking place? And, secondly, how do you know whether your DNA is mutating at an abnormal rate due to the effects of free-radicals?

Let's start with prevention. When you build up toxic reactive oxygen species in your body you have two options. Either you can nip this process in the bud so that these harmful substances are rendered innocuous, or you can incorporate your antioxidant defences to quench this free-radical fire. In order to detoxify potentially destructive chemicals, thereby rendering them harmless, you have to ensure that your liver is in top shape. Cruciferous vegetables such as broccoli, brussel sprouts, cabbage and cauliflower—all your good old favourites— and the antioxidant glutathione, occupy a central role in the liver's detoxification process. In particular, certain derivatives of cabbage metabolism called indole-3-carbinol and diindolylmethane (try saying that with a mouth full of chewing gum) have been found to be potent inducers of the liver's detoxifying mechanism, but more about that later. With regard to antioxidants, you should have some idea by now as to how you can fortify yourself. Just to refresh your memory: strawberries, red grapes, citrus fruits, apples, onions and maritime pine bark are some of the nutrients that will boost your antioxidant fortress.

Naturally you'd also be very curious to know whether free-radicals are overwhelming your antioxidant defences, as well as whether your DNA is undergoing damage and mutation. Fortunately, there is a laboratory in this country (address included at the back) that performs highly sophisticated tests that can provide you with vital information concerning your DNA status, free-radical load and antioxidant capabilities. Once you have had these tests you can make the necessary adjustments by means of the appropriate diet and nutritional supplements. This will allow you to abort any threatening developments and avert a possible disaster. Personally, I'd rather know that I had an excess of free-radicals associated with an increase in DNA mutations so that I could take action at the outset.

Once your cells have escaped this initial form of surveillance—and cancer cells being the slippery little suckers that they are, are quite adept at eluding your defences—there are still a number of aces you can play to turn the whole game around. Abnormal cells can either undergo differentiation, which means that they can change back into normal cells, or they can undergo what is called apoptosis, which is natural cell death. Again you have a whole range of very effective nutrients that are very adept at helping these two processes along. EPA and DHA, found in the oils of cold water fish such as salmon and mackerel as well as in flaxseed, canola and walnuts, are powerful differentiating agents. Soy and the herb red clover, which are rich in the phyto-oestrogens genistein and daidzein, have multi-role functions as they are able to accelerate both differentiation and apoptosis. This is why they have become such hot property in the cancer prevention arena.

So you can see that it becomes extremely difficult for any cancer to establish itself if you have enough of the right nutrients on board. It is still possible, however, for any cancer to survive at this stage, especially if the barricades are weak. Then the cancer may undergo promotion, which depends upon hormone imbalances; invasion, if the connective tissue around your cells becomes vulnerable; and finally the cancer metastasises or spreads when your immune system becomes overwhelmed. There are other intricate cellular biochemical reactions that lead to the proliferation of cancer, and it's also necessary for any growing cancer to establish its own blood supply in order to survive. All of these processes are equally subject to nutritional prevention with soy, garlic, shark cartilage, green tea, fish oil, grape seed and vitamin C being the major players.

Now let's turn our attention to the number one cancers affecting both sexes, namely prostate and breast cancer.

Preventing Prostate Cancer

The prostate is the kind of gland that remains blissfully inconspicuous until it starts to cause problems. Then it becomes a real pain in the rear end. As it so happens, that is exactly where the prostate is located, just behind the scrotum. It is a small, muscular gland, no bigger than the size of a walnut, which sits at the neck of the bladder, encircling the urethra as it carries the urine to the penis (Figure 8).

The ball game starts to get tough once the prostate increases in size, as this leads to the obstruction of the outflow of urine. This results in the symptoms that have come to be associated with prostate enlargement. These include a delay in the onset of urination, and dribbling as it ends, as well as the rather annoying inconvenience of having to get out of a warm bed to go to the toilet during the night. This is what awaits more than 50 per cent of men as they pass the halfway mark in their lives. For just over 11 per cent of men, these symptoms will herald

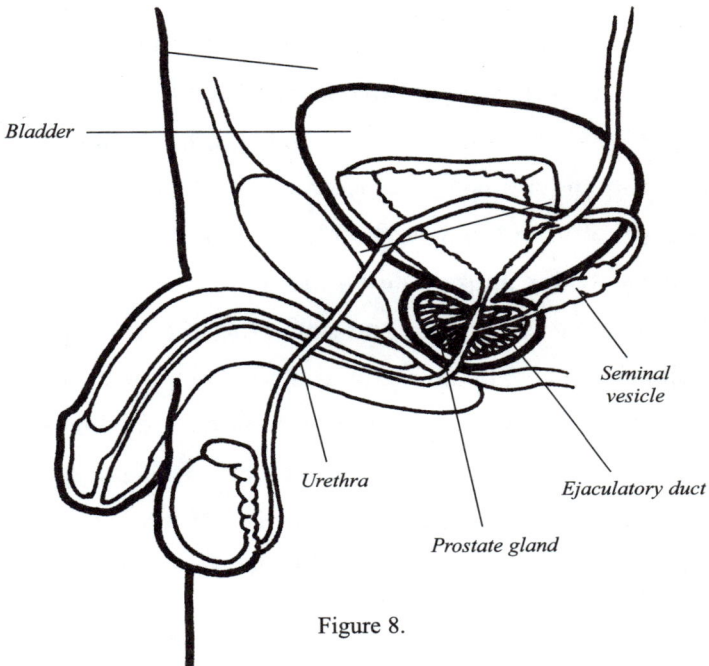

Figure 8.

the onset of prostate cancer. This is the terrible truth about this disease. A large proportion of cancers are discovered only when enlarged prostates are removed because they are becoming a nuisance. With modern-day means of surveillance via regular blood tests—which measure what is called the PSA (prostate specific antigen)—and periodic physical examinations, it is possible to pick up any change in prostate status before things start to get out of hand. However, you do not want to rely solely on these tests to tell you whether you are at risk or not. What you really want to do is look after your prostate so that you don't have to negotiate the consequences of prostate enlargement and the development of cancer. The 50 million dollar question is how do you do this?

Some of you will also be wandering whether G-d was taking a little afternoon nap when he bestowed upon the male sex the honour of having a prostate. If all it does is enlarge and get in the way, then what is the advantage of having such an annoying organ? Actually the prostate does do some good as its function is to provide lubrication, nutrition and protection for the sperm on their journey down the urethra. Sexuality is tied in with prostatic secretions, and when these start to diminish, the male sexual fire begins to smoulder. This is why males in some cultures practise contracting the pubococcygeus muscle in order to prevent the escape of semen. This is reputed to generate energy and increase lifespan. The now famous G-spot finds its home on the prostate, which, for some, is a source of much amusement.

So there are a number of reasons for doing everything you can to promote the health of your prostate. As the incidence of prostate cancer is on the increase it behoves each and every male to be especially solicitous about the wellbeing of his prostate. Diets high in animal fat, particularly red meat and dairy products, have been linked to an increased risk of developing prostate cancer (1). Scientific studies have found that the following foods and nutrients protect the prostate:

- Diets high in fruit and vegetables
- Vitamin C
- Vitamin E
- Zinc
- Phyto-oestrogens found in soy and red clover
- Selenium

- Progesterone
- Testosterone
- Cruciferous vegetables
- DHEA
- Saw Palmetto
- Melatonin
- Lycopene in tomatoes

How all these substances operate is extremely fascinating because it demonstrates the evolution of our understanding of the workings of the prostate. In order to understand why you need to incorporate the above nutrients and hormones, you need to become familiar with some key biochemical reactions in the prostate. Figure 9 demonstrates the principal hormonal pathways that take place.

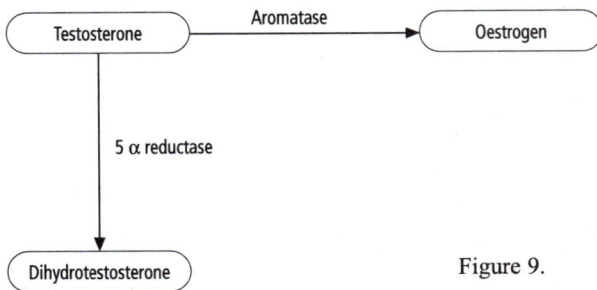

Figure 9.

As you can see, testosterone gives rise to dihydrotestosterone (DHT), a much more potent male hormone. This is achieved by means of an enzyme called 5 alpha reductase. Testosterone also forms oestrogen by means of an enzyme called aromatase. The core wisdom in this biochemical conundrum is to achieve a state of balance. You want just the right amount of DHT, you don't want too much oestrogen, and you want to maintain your testosterone at optimal levels. It's not as complicated as it sounds and there are blood tests, or, even better, salivary hormone assays, that will guide you along the way.

The above substances are critical because they influence the expression of the above key enzymes. To prevent the conversion of testosterone to oestrogen, which current wisdom dictates is bad for your prostate and may lead to the development of cancer, you need to block the action of the enzyme aromatase. The phyto-oestrogens found in soy and red clover will achieve this end. The amount of aromatase you have in your body is proportional to the amount of fat you are carrying, which means that it's not a good idea to be sporting too much extra adipose tissue. Zinc deficiency will also increase the activity of aromatase. If you consume lots of sunflower and pumpkin seeds topped up with lashings of that well known aphrodisiac, oyster, you will increase your zinc levels, thereby inhibiting the activity of aromatase. Cruciferous vegetables such as cabbage, broccoli and cauliflower and their metabolic by-products indole-3-carbinol and diindolylmethane, ensure that any oestrogen lurking in your system is converted to a harmless form of this hormone that won't affect your prostate.

Zinc and DHEA will boost your levels of testosterone if these are low. The other process that you need to control is the conversion of testosterone to DHT, as too much DHT is not considered beneficial. To suppress the conversion of testosterone to DHT you have to inhibit the action of enzyme 5 alpha-reductase. Zinc and the phyto-oestrogens will serve you in this area, as will the herb saw palmetto. The hormone progesterone is also reputed to reduce 5 alpha-reductase activity. A welcome side-effect of this approach may be the regeneration of hair growth as excess DHT is thought to contribute to baldness.

Fruits and vegetables are considered important because they are rich in antioxidants that are known to be cancer protective. This is why vitamins C and E, melatonin and the mineral selenium are all so essential, as they markedly enhance your antioxidant defences.

The phyto-oestrogens found in soy and red clover are so vital, not only because they modulate the levels of your various hormones, but also because they suppress the expression of growth factors located in your prostate that are thought to encourage the development of cancer cells. Lycopene, found in tomatoes, is thought to operate in a similar fashion. If you want to absorb maximum amounts of lycopene when you consume tomatoes, try adding olive oil, as certain fats are known to enhance the bio-availability of lycopene. Phyto-oestrogens also block the effects of excess oestrogen on your prostate. If any cancer cells manage to elude these powerful nutrients, they will still have a rocky road ahead of them. Phyto-oestrogens prevent cancer cells from establishing their own blood supply and they prohibit the spread of cancer. This is why oriental populations are so wise in making soy products a large staple of their diet.

For those of you who have been warned off DHEA because it is supposed to stimulate the development of cancer in the prostate, it appears that the opposite is true. Studies show that

DHEA levels in men with prostate cancer are lower than DHEA levels in men who do not have prostate cancer (2). Furthermore, a number of studies bear testament to the fact that DHEA actually inhibits the growth of prostate cancer cells, and the higher the concentration the greater the inhibition of growth. DHEA only becomes a problem if you already have too much testosterone in your body as it will then be shunted down the oestrogen pathway, which will have adverse consequences.

By adopting a diet that optimises the health of your prostate, together with the judicious modulation of hormones and the right nutrient supplementation, you can preserve your sexual vitality and avoid any of the debilitating effects of prostate cancer. When you commit yourself to this program it is probably a good idea to seek the guidance of a knowledgeable health practitioner as you will need regular monitoring of your hormone levels (including melatonin and DHEA) as well as your PSA.

Preventing Breast Cancer

Breast cancer is by far the most common cancer diagnosed in women. The alarming fact is that the incidence of breast cancer is skyrocketing. In the USA from 1980 to 1987, the number of breast cancer cases rose by 32 per cent (3). Today, a woman's lifetime risk of acquiring breast cancer is one in eight (4).

The cause for this epidemic is thought to result from a considerable over-exposure to the hormone oestrogen. Earlier onset of menarche, reduction in child-bearing years, reliance on the oral contraceptive pill and hormone replacement therapy later in life lead to a constant stream of oestrogen stimulation. This is exacerbated by environmental exposure to pesticides, herbicides and plastics, which result in a build-up of false oestrogens, or xeno-oestrogens as they are called, in the body. These xeno-oestrogens are able to mimic the effects of oestrogen, which adds to the problem of a steady state of oestrogen activity. Excess body mass and a diet high in saturated animal fat will also enhance the presence of oestrogen, further compounding the risk. It's important to establish that oestrogen doesn't actually cause breast cancer. It merely encourages abnormal cells to multiply, somewhat like a coach spurring a team on to even greater achievements. Only in this case the result is not a team victory, but rather a catastrophe. This is why you have to marshal your resources so that the coach is not allowed much of a peak at the game.

To develop abnormal cells in the first place, your DNA has to mutate unremittingly. For women, an antioxidant-rich diet found in fruit and vegetables is essential. If you are going to prevent your DNA from mutating, you need to stop those pesky free-radicals dead in their tracks, and there's no better way to do it than by having a healthy supply of antioxidants ready and waiting. The same vitamins and minerals that are protective to the male prostate are equally important for breast cancer prevention. These include:

- Vitamin C
- Vitamin E
- Zinc
- Selenium

Add the carotenoids found in carrots, apricots, spinach, pumpkin and sweet potatoes to your antioxidant team as these will also decrease the risk of breast cancer. If you really want to go for broke, it is a wise choice to augment your diet with the other powerful antioxidants such as:

- Green tea
- Pine bark extract
- Red grape extract
- Beetroot juice

The hormone melatonin is an equally vital component of your antioxidant arsenal. There is now solid evidence that in addition to its impressive antioxidant capabilities, melatonin is able to suppress the proliferation of human breast cancer cells while increasing the expression of a very significant gene called p53 (5). The p53 gene is known to inhibit the development of cancer whereas the mutation of another gene called BRCA1 leads to the development of cancer.

It's probably a good idea to touch briefly on the genetics of cancer as I'm sure there will be those of you who will be worried about all the research currently focused on the genetic causes of this disease. In the majority of cases, studies indicate that breast cancer is not a genetically inherited disease. Most women diagnosed with breast cancer do not have abnormal genes, although if you have a family history of this illness the likelihood of your contracting cancer does increase. Breast cancer is predominantly caused by factors that you can influence, which is tremendously encouraging. As I've mentioned before, even bad genes can be nullified by good lifestyle practices.

Once you've neutralised the effects of free-radicals you then have to modulate the effects of oestrogen on your breasts. Modulate is a really good term because what it means is that you want just the right amount of oestrogen—not too much and not too little. It also implies that you have control over the outcome of events. You have to start by preserving your best weight, something that a lot of women have a problem with as they get older. The more you put on weight the more you place yourself at the mercy of having an over-supply of oestrogen in your body. I encourage all my female patients to enjoy a variety of exercise activities including aerobics, yoga, walking, stretching and weight training, which is especially important as it preserves your lean muscle mass. I'm not suggesting that you have to be the next Ms Universe, but you have to get out there and become active.

Next, you have to go easy on the alcohol consumption. More than two gasses of red wine per night places an added strain on your liver, which has to metabolise oestrogen so that it can be eliminated. A sluggish liver will increase the amount of oestrogen in your body, which may be harmful.

Then you need to have an adequate supply of the phyto-oestrogens derived from soy and red clover, which operate very similarly to the way they do in the male body. They block the effects of excess oestrogen and they also convert oestrogen to a less potent form of this hormone called oestriol, which you will learn about in the chapter on HRT. Phyto-oestrogens also stimulate differentiation and apoptosis, two processes that ensure that abnormal cells die a natural death rather than multiplying as cancer cells.

The other major nutrients that promote a beneficial outcome in the metabolism of oestrogen are found in cruciferous vegetables. These vegetables possess unique phyto-nutrient constituents called indole-3-carbinol and diindolylmethane, which were mentioned earlier as part of the prostate prevention program. What they do is to favourably modify oestrogen to harmless forms of this hormone called 2-hydroxy and 2-methoxyoestrogens. These metabolites have been labelled the 'good oestrogens' as they have the power to prevent any abnormal cells from proliferating, while eliminating any damaged or abnormal cells that have accumulated in the body (6). The phyto-nutrients in cruciferous vegetables are able to generate the 'good oestrogens' by promoting detoxification pathways that exist in the liver. Without these nutrients, 'bad oestrogens' accumulate in the form of 16-hydroxyoestrone. These 'bad oestrogens' are associated with higher rates of breast cancer (7). As it is not possible to obtain sufficient amounts of indole-3-carbinol and diindolylmethane from the diet alone, it is necessary to take these in supplement form. The beauty of these nutrients is that they allow you to entertain the possibility of taking HRT with the knowledge that you can minimise the risks of developing breast cancer.

The Cancer Preventing Diet

This diet should contain fruit and vegetables in abundance, preferably those that are organic so that you limit the effects of pesticides and herbicides. Animal fats, which have been found to boost the levels of the 'bad oestrogens', can be substituted with the fats found in fish and olive oil, which produce more of the 'good oestrogens' identified as the 2-hydroxymetabolites. Add to this a liberal assortment of antioxidant nutrients, including vitamins A, C and E and the minerals zinc and selenium, plus some of the other more potent antioxidants such as green tea and red grape extract. Finally, have a good supply of the phyto-oestrogens found in soy and red clover combined with the phyto-nutrients in cruciferous vegetables at the ready, and cancer cells beware! This dietary approach is a unisex one and it offers you a veritable fortress that any cancer would find very hard to breach.

No cancer cell is going to catch me

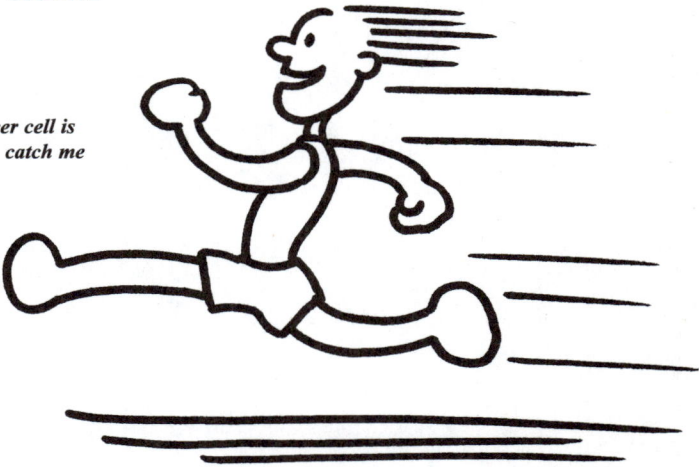

Key Points To Remember

The following nutrients and hormones are of paramount importance in your cancer preventing program:

- Fruit and vegetables
- Vitamin A
- Vitamin C
- Vitamin E

- Zinc
- Selenium
- Green tea
- Red grape extract
- Melatonin
- DHEA
- The phyto-oestrogens in soy and red clover
- The phyto-nutrients in cruciferous vegetables

CHAPTER 7

The Change
Of Life

The Change
Of Life

*O*F ALL THE ANTI-AGEING CHALLENGES ENCOUNTERED IN LIFE, menopause, in my opinion, is the most difficult to deal with. You can say all you like about liberation and the gaining of wisdom, but in my experience this is a very difficult time for women. Menopause is a time when a clear biological change takes place, and decisions need to be made about the best way to deal with the immediate symptoms and the long-term consequences of hormone deficiency. Hormone replacement therapy (HRT), the natural alternatives, or simply carrying on with life are the choices that face the fairer sex as they pass into this transitional phase. Men don't have such an obvious biological transition to deal with and they don't always understand exactly what women have to go through. This is one of the reasons I find it so difficult to counsel women with regard to this period. Therefore, when I inform my patients of the risks of osteoporosis and heart disease, which are considerable for post-menopausal women, I feel like I am preaching. Unfortunately there is still a lot of confusing and conflicting information about the best way to deal with menopause. Many women still view HRT with considerable suspicion. Professor Maida Taylor, from the Department of Reproductive Sciences at the University of California, San Francisco, informs us that only 10 to 25 per cent of menopausal women take HRT (1). Of prescriptions written for HRT only 50 per cent are filled, and after one year, only 40 per cent of women persist with HRT. According to Professor Taylor, most women reject HRT for three major reasons:

1. FEAR OF MALIGNANCY

For a large proportion of women, HRT is still associated with cancer, especially that of the breast. The very thought that this remains a possibility, however much this is unsubstantiated by scientific fact, is enough to put most women off the notion of taking HRT. Cancer is associated with crippling disfigurements, horrible treatments and the possibility of a slow, lingering, painful death. Despite the fact that the statistics for osteoporotic fractures and heart disease far exceed that of cancer, it is an uphill battle to convince women that their fears are unfounded.

2. SIDE EFFECTS

Most women have the impression that HRT is more trouble than it is worth. Having negotiated the indignities of regular periods for longer than they care to remember, the last thing that women want is to endure more of the same. Because of their experiences with the oral contraceptive pill, many women believe that HRT promotes weight gain. Although the textbooks claim that this is not the case and the facts indicate that HRT users are no fatter than non-users, for many women this is a very real problem. Breast pain occurs in a substantial number of women who are on HRT. Some are frightened by this experience as it suggests cancer and this often stops women from continuing to take hormones.

3. THE IDEA THAT MENOPAUSE IS A DEFICIENCY DISEASE

With the changing way that women view their health, most do not like to view menopause as a disease that needs indefinite medical management. This would mean that they no longer have control of their health, and that they would need to depend on an establishment that is not always sympathetic to their needs. It is for these reasons that non-medical alternatives have become so attractive to women.

Non-medical treatments for the symptoms of menopause are seen to be harmless, natural and side-effect-free, allowing women to make choices that can only have positive outcomes. When medical authorities tell us that women on HRT have 60 per cent less heart attacks, 20 to 40 per cent fewer deaths from cancer, and live on average 4.2 years longer than women not on HRT, these facts fall mostly on deaf ears (2).

To achieve a state of balance, which I believe is one of the cornerstones of any anti-ageing program, it is necessary to present all the facts as they stand at the present time and let you make an informed choice as to how you would like to proceed. The best place to start is with the major hormonal agents in this ongoing saga, oestrogen and progesterone.

Oestrogen

Oestrogen is the hormone responsible for the development of secondary sexual characteristics in the maturing female. The growth and development of the vagina, the enlargement of the breasts and the formation of the typical female body contours are due to the effects of oestrogen. Oestrogen is produced predominantly during the first part of the menstrual cycle, during which time it stimulates the lining of the uterus to become thicker. This is intended to make the womb receptive to the fertilised ovum. Oestrogen also encourages breast cells to proliferate.

Your body produces three predominant forms of oestrogen: oestradiol, which forms 10 to 20 per cent of circulating oestrogen and is regarded as the strongest of the oestrogens as far as breast cell stimulation is concerned; oestrone, which makes up a further 10 to 20 per cent of circulating oestrogen and is the predominant hormone secreted post-menopausally; and oestriol, which comprises 60 to 80 per cent of total oestrogen and is secreted mostly during pregnancy.

Oestrogen is the hormone that has undergone a roller-coaster ride ever since Dr John Lee, who has pioneered work on the relationship between progesterone and menopause, and others started talking about the problems of oestrogen excess. While oestrogen is good for the brain, heart, skin and the skeletal system, having too much of this hormone places the breasts and the uterus at risk. Oestrogen over-stimulation is associated with PMS, water retention, headaches, breast tenderness, fatigue and a host of other maladies. Dr Lee has even gone so far as to suggest that menopause is really about progesterone deficiency. He believes we have been missing the boat when it comes to dealing appropriately with this transitional stage.

Progesterone

Progesterone is the hormone that is synthesised mostly during the second half of the menstrual cycle. Progesterone's role is to ensure that the endometrium (lining of the uterus) is maintained so that the fertilised ovum can survive. During pregnancy, progesterone production increases to protect the foetus and it does this by preventing any untimely shedding of the uterine lining. If you refer to Figure 4 in Chapter 2, you will notice that aside from the ovaries, progesterone is also formed in the adrenal glands and is the precursor of all the other hormones produced in these glands. It is therefore able to exert some influence over blood sugar control, salt regulation and the activity of the sex steroid hormones. Dr Lee is of the opinion that progesterone has a wide range of beneficial actions. Stimulating elimination via the kidneys, normalising blood clotting and reversing depression are just some of the advantages of adequate progesterone production. It is when we examine menopause that we discover the influential role that oestrogen and progesterone play, not all of which is agreed upon by the experts.

Menopausal Systems

For most women, hot flushes, night sweats, vaginal dryness and mood swings herald the onset of a rather unpleasant period that they could happily do without. Despite the fact that women are wary of HRT, Premarin—which is a synthetic form of oestrogen—remains one of the hottest selling drugs, outstripping remedies as popular as Zantac and Prozac. In the USA, 22 million prescriptions were written for Premarin during 1996 (3). Of all the different approaches used to treat menopausal symptoms, conventional HRT remains the most successful, achieving a strike rate in the range of 80 to 90 per cent. Non-hormonal measures can only boast a 30 to 60 per cent average (4).

The downside of HRT is the side-effects. Because the kinds of oestrogen and progesterone used are mostly synthetic, and oestrogen is incorporated in its most potent form as oestradiol, women taking HRT may find themselves substituting one symptom for another. Breast swelling, irritability, irregular bleeding, bloating and depression are some of the consequences of taking HRT. However, local experts reassure us that these side-effects are soon resolved (5). The real difficulty revolves around the incorporation of such a powerful hormone as oestradiol, which is known to affect the cells of the breasts. This is why Dr Jonathon Wright, who has popularised the use of natural hormone replacement therapy creams, advocates the use of oestriol in its natural form, which is a milder variety of oestrogen (6). This has been found to be as effective as the stronger oestrogens in relieving menopausal symptoms without the troublesome side-effects. Dr Lee, the progesterone expert, concurs with this and also suggests that the focus on oestrogen deficiency has been ill-conceived. He maintains that we should really recognise the hormone that undergoes the most dramatic decline in menopause—progesterone. Dr Lee claims that his experience with giving natural progesterone in the form of a cream is a very useful way of dealing with the symptoms of menopause without any adverse consequences.

Asian women eat a lot of soy-based foods that are rich in phyto-oestrogens, and they also suffer from very few menopausal symptoms, especially hot flushes. Studies that have utilised various sources of phyto-oestrogens have demon-strated a reasonable reduction in menopausal symptoms with these nutrients (7). The herb black cohosh has yielded similar results. The bottom line is that alternative treatments, while being less effective, are far more user friendly. Drs Wright and Lee claim that the natural creams are the way to go, but their work still needs to be substantiated by a more extensive research base.

Osteoporosis

This is one of the most underrated challenges that women have to deal with. More than one third of women will sustain a fracture due to osteoporosis at some stage of their lives and the consequences can result in a long period of disability. As for the treatment of menopausal symptoms, HRT remains the gold standard in the management of this condition. No other form of therapy has undergone the trials that HRT has endured to prove its worth. The good news is that oestrogen use by women, starting at the age of 60 and continuing for nine years, leads to just as much bone preservation as that which results from oestrogen supplementation from the outset of menopause (8).

However, the key lies in looking after your bones before menopause sets in. Peak bone mass occurs around the age of 16 to 25, after which bone density gradually declines. Although genes contribute significantly to the development of osteoporosis, lifestyle factors can influence the promotion of healthy bones. Cigarette smoking, alcohol abuse and diets high in animal protein, salt and caffeine will do your bones no favours. A vegetarian and grain-based diet will create an alkaline environment within the cells of your body, which is an optimal medium for effective bone mineralisation.

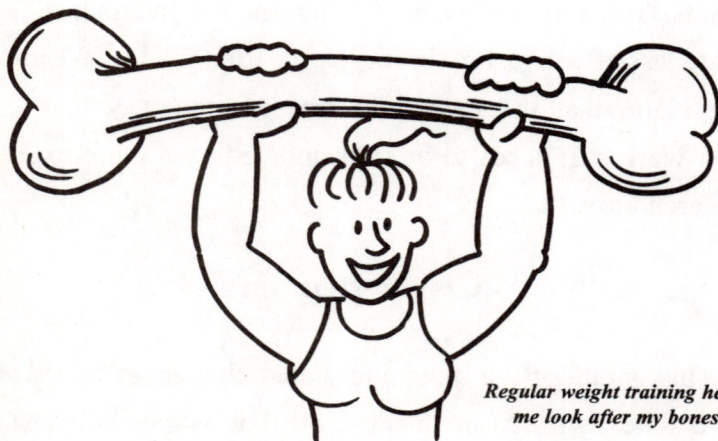

Regular weight training helps me look after my bones

Regular exercise is crucial for building strong bones. Studies have shown that weight training is the best way to prevent osteoporosis. What you need to do is to commence a weight-training program with progressive increments in the weights that you lift. This will strengthen your muscles and bones concurrently. If this proposition sounds unattractive to you, I am not suggesting that you have to become Arnold Schwarzenegger. All you have to do is commence a modest program and slowly increase your efforts. You will become more toned, which will make you the envy of all of your friends, and your bones will appreciate your efforts.

There are certain nutrients that are essential for effective bone mineralisation:

CALCIUM: This is a well recognised bone nutrient, and, as 90 per cent of bone mass accumulates by the age of 25, calcium intake needs to be sufficient during this early period. I am not swayed by the Dairy Board's insistence that milk is the best source of calcium. Lactose intolerance makes it difficult for some women to digest milk and the casein in milk binds proteins whereby they are lost from the body. Nuts, green vegetables and soy products are excellent sources of calcium. Microcrystalline hydroxyapatite is a highly bioavailable form of calcium found in bonemeal, which has been found to have promising effects on bone mineralisation. Oestrogen improves the gastrointestinal absorption of calcium, which diminishes after the age of 70. Adequate calcium intake slows the loss of bone after menopause and augments the positive effects of exercise and oestrogen on bone mass (9).

MAGNESIUM: Some authorities consider this nutrient to be as important as calcium for the effective mineralisation of bone. Magnesium increases calcium absorption and facilitates its role in bone building by activating vitamin D. Vitamin D is required for calcium assimilation into bones and teeth. Magnesium is found in dark green vegetables, nuts and legumes—similar sources to those of calcium.

BORON: This is not an essential nutrient, however, this mineral does reduce the urinary excretion of calcium and magnesium as well as increasing the serum concentration of oestrogen and testosterone.

PHYTO-OESTROGENS: As well as having a lower incidence of menopausal symptoms, Asian women have a low prevalence of osteoporosis and hip fractures. We know that the Asian diet is rich in phyto-oestrogens. While there has not been a numerous array of studies to substantiate these findings, one study did show that when post-menopausal women were given a soy protein-enriched diet for six months, their bone mineral content increased as compared with that of a group of women given a milk-based diet (10). Ipriflavone, a synthetic type of phyto-oestrogen, has been found to prevent bone loss and stimulate collagen synthesis in bone.

The Hormones

When we talk about building healthy bones and preventing osteoporosis, hormones remain the critical influence. As I've indicated, the only long-term studies performed to date show that HRT in the form of synthetic oestrogen and progestogen (synthetic progesterone) remains the current reliable inhibitor of osteoporosis. This has stimulated a huge amount of opposition from doctors like Lee and Wright who contend that progesterone in its natural form is what we should really be focusing on. Dr Lee claims that it is the decline in progesterone, which is far more dramatic than oestrogen at the time of the menopause, that accounts for the acceleration in bone loss. Progesterone, says Dr Lee, stops bone loss while stimulating the growth of new bone, which he asserts oestrogen does not do. In fact, this is not true. Oestrogen has been found to do exactly the same. To verify the role that progesterone is purported to play, Dr Lee administered natural progesterone derived from the herb wild yam to 100 patients, which they applied to their skin in cream form. During a three-year period, Dr Lee demonstrated an average increase in bone density of 14 per cent in the lumbar spine (lower back), with the greatest improvements noted in those with the worst bone density at the commencement of the trial. As these results are clearly impressive, studies are now underway to test these findings, but aside from individual cases that support Dr Lee's work, there is no other experimental evidence to verify his results.

I suggest that if you do opt to take the natural route, have your bone density checked to make sure you are benefiting from your program. I advise all my patients to supplement their diets with phyto-oestrogens, either derived from soy or red clover, together with microcrystalline hydroxyapatite, magnesium and boron. I also whip them into shape by encouraging them to start an exercise regime that includes weight training.

HRT And Cancer

The scourge of cancer hangs over HRT like a dark cloud. Of all the factors that dampen women's enthusiasm for HRT, the possibility of developing cancer is by far the strongest. The likelihood of developing endometrial cancer is eliminated when progesterone, either in its natural or synthetic form, is added to oestrogen supplementation. The real issue concerns breast cancer. Here authorities are divided on the relative risks. Australian experts reassure us that long-term HRT users only have a moderate chance of developing breast cancer. Of women who take HRT for five years, an extra two out of 1000 will develop breast cancer, and, after a 10-year period, this figure increases to six out of 1000. At a recent presentation to the American Academy of Anti-Ageing Medicine, American authority Dr Shari Lieberman warned that the figure for women who are on HRT for five years is closer to 30 per cent, which is certainly different from the way our experts interpret the statistics. Others confirm that these averages escalate if there is a family history of breast cancer.

Dr Wright, who advocates the use of natural oestrogen creams in a book entitled Natural Hormone Replacement, suggests that oestriol may be a better option as it is less stimulating to breast tissue and may actually protect the breast and the endometrium from the stimulatory effects of the other oestrogens, oestradiol and oestrone. He cites evidence to indicate that women who develop breast cancer have lower levels of oestriol than those who don't. Asian women who have a low incidence of breast cancer have higher levels of oestriol compared to their American counterparts. Dr Wright, who is an avid fan of Dr Lee's work, also supports the use of natural progesterone cream, using experimental evidence to show that progesterone inhibits the multiplication of breast cancer cells.

As far as oestriol is concerned, other studies demonstrate that this hormone is not as harmless as it is made out to be. Professor Maida Taylor presents evidence to show that in post-menopausal women, high levels of oestriol in the bloodstream correlate with high levels of breast cancer, however, in pre-menopausal women, the higher the level of oestriol the lower the incidence of breast cancer (11).

Studies performed on natural progesterone also bring its credibility into question. Recent research performed at the Sydney Menopause Centre found no evidence that natural progesterone cream decreased the proliferation of cells lining the endometrium, which is the wall of the uterus. This study suggests that if progesterone was absorbed from the skin, the amount was not sufficient to have an effect on the endometrium.

What are you supposed to make of all this conflicting evidence? Who do you listen to—the local experts or their American colleagues? Is conventional HRT dangerous and are natural hormone creams beneficial? There is no easy answer to all these questions and my heart goes out to all the women faced with these dilemmas. My impressions are that we still have a lot to learn about natural hormone creams and that more research needs to be done before their efficacy can be determined. What I do is utilise these creams and then monitor their presence by means of blood tests and salivary hormone assays before and after treatment. Salivary hormone assays are definitely more useful as these give a more accurate picture of the levels of free hormones in the body, but unfortunately these tests cannot give you a breakdown of the three different oestrogens—oestradiol, oestrone and oestriol. Incidentally, what Dr Wright does is to prescribe all three oestrogens in their natural ratios in the form of a cream called Triest, and I have recently instituted a similar regimen in my practice as he has a wealth of experience behind him. Dr Wright might just live up to his name.

I also advise all my patients about the cancer protective diet and the relevant nutrient supplements, according to the protocol listed in Chapter 6.

Heart Disease

You have already learned about the benefits that oestrogen can have on the cardiovascular system in Chapter 4. Just to give your memory a little jolt, oestrogen reduces the accumulation of fibrinogen and lipoprotein (a), which are connected with heart disease. Oestrogen also inhibits the effects of homocysteine and counteracts the presence of raised insulin levels, both of which initiate cardiovascular disease. Oestrogen increases HDL and reduces LDL. You will remember that these accolades are not shared by oestrogen alone, as experimental evidence shows that progesterone may be equally implicated in the prevention of heart disease. I also indicated that for some there still remains a question mark over the impressive effects that HRT demonstrates in promoting cardiovascular health. The highly reputable Framingham Heart Study, which analysed the connection between HRT use and heart disease in an extensive population group over a protracted period, found no advantage in oestrogen supplementation (12). It is important to appreciate that this study was performed over 13 years ago and we have discovered more about heart disease since then. Nevertheless it does add to the balance that I mentioned earlier. As you now realise, the evidence for and against HRT is not always black and white.

Senility And Alzheimer's Disease

Finally, an area to get unequivocally enthusiastic about. As you recall HRT and especially oestrogen have a significant impact on the genesis of Alzheimer's disease. Low oestrogen levels are associated with the onset of Alzheimer's, and oestrogen may delay or even prevent the onset of this destructive illness. Oestrogen may ameliorate some of the mental symptoms in women who have already developed Alzheimer's. In women, the incidence of Alzheimer's disease increases dramatically after the age of 65 so that by the time they reach 80 there is a 40 per cent chance of contracting this tragic illness. Like all degenerative diseases, Alzheimer's takes a long time to manifest so it is important not to wait for any obvious signs of mental deterioration before commencing oestrogen supplementation. The difficulty is that we don't yet have a reliable method for predicting who is at risk, which means that every woman should seriously consider taking oestrogen as a means of prevention.

For those who are tossing up between conventional HRT and the alternative modalities, Professor David Purdie of the Centre for Metabolic Bone Disease in Hull, England, may influence your decision. He is a firm endorser of HRT. As far as preventing osteoporosis is concerned, Professor Purdie insists that oestrogen is the key to maintaining strong bones. Remove oestrogen, says Professor Purdie, and bone loss outstrips bone formation and bones get weaker. With regard to the heart, Professor Purdie informs us that oestrogen is responsible for the synthesis of a substance called nitric oxide, which allows blood to flow easily and freely through the blood vessels. Loss of oestrogen promotes atherogenesis, which is the blockage of blood vessels, ultimately resulting in heart attacks.

Professor Purdie also endorses oestrogen's role in reducing the incidence of Alzheimer's disease, a factor that desperately needs to be acknowledged due to the increased frequency of this illness in women.

Exciting new studies cited by Professor Purdie that document oestrogen's part in preventing bowel cancer, inhibiting the formation of cataracts, and modulating the expression of such auto-immune diseases as rheumatoid arthritis and multiple sclerosis, provide additional evidence of oestrogen's worth.

Professor Purdie claims that 21st century medicine will see HRT evolve to address the specific losses incurred by women at menopause, and that this form of medicine will become far more precise. In particular, he mentions a new range of HRT drugs called selective oestrogen receptor modifiers (SERMS).

What SERMS do is target specific areas of the body. A prototype of this approach is the drug called Raloxifene, which predominantly affects the bones and the heart. Raloxifene inhibits osteoporosis and has no adverse effects on breast tissue. Unfortunately however, its bone-sparing powers do not match up with those of HRT and it has side-effects including hot flushes and leg cramps.

To recap, in the one corner we have conventional HRT, which has scientifically proven benefits on the heart, mind and skeletal structure. We also discover that the bowel, eyes and immune system are added benefactors. To balance this we have the possibility of cancer, however slight, looming in the background, together with all those detractors who claim that HRT is not what it is cracked up to be. And in the other corner we have the alternative treatments, which include the natural creams, herbs and phyto-oestrogens. These modalities appear to be far more attractive to women, but the downside is that they do not always have the backing of solid scientific evidence.

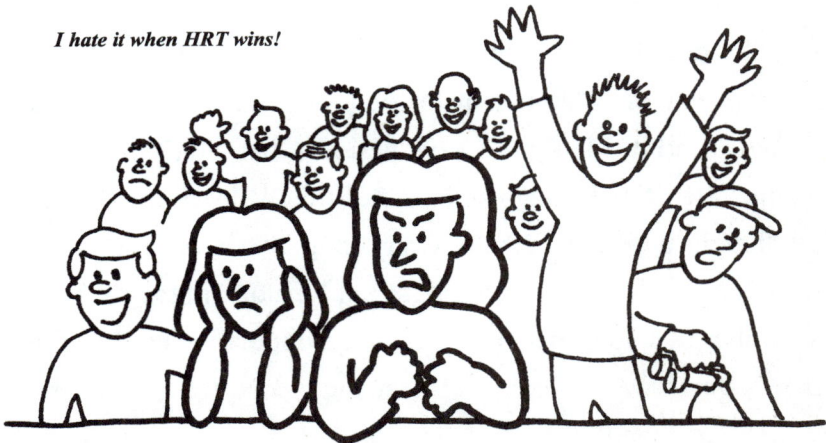

I hate it when HRT wins!

So what do I advise my female patients to do? My personal bias is to choose natural treatments. However, the evidence with regard to osteoporosis and Alzheimer's disease is pretty compelling in favour of HRT. I tend to present all the options and then evaluate risk factors on an individual basis. If the bone density indicates that osteoporosis is present and the threat of heart disease is also a reality based on the relevant blood tests, then HRT has to be entertained as a mode of therapy. I monitor all patients regularly to assess the efficacy of the approach they have adopted. I would like to believe that the natural treatments do make a difference, but I am also aware of the necessity to check this out both subjectively and objectively. As I view anti-ageing from a holistic perspective, I try not to evaluate the menopausal transition in isolation. Instead I see it as a time to focus on all the other health issues mentioned in this book. Cultivating optimal health means that you need to service your being in totality.

The Male Transition

If the two sexes are supposed to come from different planets then they are also meant to rotate in a radically different biological orbit. Men don't have periods, they don't procreate and they don't go through a change of life. At least this is what we thought until now. Just as everything else is turning on its head, it appears that women might not be alone in their plight. A number of studies performed on large populations of healthy men have shown a marked rise in impotence to over 50 per cent in men aged 60 to 70 (13). Some statistics even indicate that one in every four adult males experiences some form of erectile dysfunction, as impotence is now called.

The stocks of testosterone, the once mighty male hormone, appear to be plummeting. So much so that a term has been invented for this decline. Andropause, which is the male answer to menopause, is now being viewed by some experts as a legitimate condition caused by diminishing levels of testosterone. It goes without saying that andropause is not without its detractors. They claim that hormonal levels in men are variable throughout life and it is not accurate to describe a male menopause. But this hasn't stopped the andropause specialists from enumerating the features that typify this transition.

The Characteristics Of Andropause

If you are between the ages of 45 and 60 and you are experiencing a cluster of the following signs, you may just be going through andropause.

- Increasing fatigue
- Excessive sweating
- Irritability and mood swings
- Depression
- Impotence
- Flabby muscles and weight gain
- Anxiety and decreased assertiveness
- Skin wrinkling and the development of grey hair
- Aches and pains in the muscles and joints

When we examine the natural progression of testosterone, we find that it peaks in the late teens and declines gradually from the age of 30. After 40, this decline proceeds at the rate of one per cent per annum. Although there are some men who will not conform to this pattern, for a reasonable majority, this is what awaits them. However, to explain such a mass reduction in potency, something more has to be draining this huge reservoir of male hormone. Proponents of the andropause theory place the blame fairly and squarely on the shoulders of 20th century living. They claim that andropause can be explained if we focus on the consequences of modern-day living, which result in a reduction of testosterone.

1. TOO MUCH OESTROGEN

Men are bathed in a sea of oestrogen, which is caused by environmental contamination with man-made chemicals such as DDT, PCB and other pesticides that are found in the soil. These false oestrogens, or xeno-oestrogens as they are called, find a haven in our bodies when we ingest the produce of the poisoned soil. In males, xeno-oestrogens diminish the potency of testosterone and reduce sperm counts. Men with high oestrogen levels will not be gold-medal winners in the sexual Olympics. A way around this is to eat organic fruit and vegetables, which lessens the exposure to these nasty hormones, but you have to remember that these chemicals are capable of hanging around for a long time and it will require a very conscious environmental policy to eradicate this threat.

2. FREE-RADICAL DAMAGE

These toxins have a pervasive effect on all our hormones and testosterone is no exception. Free-radicals and heavy metals such as lead, arsenic, mercury and cadmium can reduce testosterone levels.

3. STRESS

Living in the fast lane erodes sex drive. The negative effects of living in the urban jungle don't do testosterone any good. Men who are intense, competitive and driven tend to have an increased production of the stress hormone cortisol. When the body produces too much cortisol then DHEA, the adrenal hormone that generates testosterone, suffers. Testosterone levels then go down. Women beware: men who are high achievers and materially well endowed may not deliver when it comes to the antics of the bedroom.

4. LOW CHOLESTEROL

Testosterone is made from cholesterol. We can't do without cholesterol and yet the pharmaceutical industry would have us believe that this essential nutrient is some type of gigantic menace, reeking cardiovascular havoc wherever it has the audacity to set foot. Studies indicate that older people benefit from having above normal cholesterol levels, and that the overzealous lowering of cholesterol may be doing us more harm than good.

5. ALCOHOL AND OBESITY

Although these don't always go hand in hand, regular drinking does encourage the kind of eating behaviour that may lead to weight gain. Initial alcohol consumption raises testosterone levels, however, with time and increasing exposure to alcohol, testosterone production diminishes.

One of the consequences of obesity is insulin resistance, which has adverse metabolic effects on other hormones. One of these hormones is DHEA, the production of which dwindles when insulin levels escalate, usually taking testosterone along with it.

6. INADEQUATE NUTRITION

One of the nutrients that is needed to build testosterone is zinc. Zinc deficiency is almost endemic in our society and it gets worse as we grow older. Consuming foods that are high in zinc such as nuts, seeds, legumes and oysters, is one of the ways to preserve normal testosterone.

7. MELATONIN AND THYROID HORMONE

Just to show you how connected your hormonal system really is, low melatonin is associated with reduced testosterone levels. When melatonin declines with age, the pituitary produces less adrenocorticotrophic hormone (ACTH). ACTH has the job of firing up your adrenals to produce DHEA. When ACTH levels drop, so do DHEA levels, and you know what this entails for testosterone. Likewise, waning thyroid hormone compromises testosterone.

So men are up against it, and testosterone, which should be the pride and joy of all the male members of the species, is being well and truly humbled. Although the process is different and the causes aren't exactly the same, men now find them-selves in a similar predicament to women. If you scrutinise the features of andropause, you will realise that they resemble those of menopause in many respects, in which case we need to consider HRT for men just as we do for women.

In many anti-ageing centres, HRT for men is becoming a reality and not without justification. You see, testosterone is a vitally important hormone and it does most males a power of good. It all starts at puberty when testosterone assumes responsibility for the development of secondary sexual characteristics such as the deepening of the voice, the growth of the genitalia, the sprouting of body hair and the production of sperm. Testosterone also promotes muscle and bone growth, and in all these functions, it is fulfilling its androgenic destiny, ie.— making a man a man. Testosterone is considered to be the most powerful stimulator of mitochondrial function. If we go about our daily activities with an abundance of energy, then we have testosterone to thank for providing us with this essential commodity. Healthy bone maintenance is sustained by testosterone, which means that when testosterone declines, men are faced with the reality of developing osteoporosis. This is not solely a woman's problem. A healthy libido is dependent on testosterone, and prostatic wellbeing is now attributed to adequate testosterone levels. The heart and the immune system are positively influenced by normal levels of testosterone.

It's a crying shame then that we are witnessing the ongoing decline of this once mighty hormone. The obvious way to manage this is to introduce the same approach that we have been utilising for women for years—enter HRT for men. Testosterone replacement therapy is now a routine event in anti-ageing clinics around the globe, and to date the results are impressive. This type of therapy can have a significant impact on andropause by reversing all the negative features detailed earlier and replacing them with positive outcomes. The time has come for men to seriously entertain the necessity for hormone replacement therapy in the form of testosterone. Let's have a look at what can be achieved with this type of treatment.

Testosterone Replacement Therapy

1. THE ANABOLIC EFFECTS OF TESTOSTERONE

Anabolic means to build up, and as far as the body goes, testosterone has anabolic effects on muscle and bone. This has been well demonstrated in older men, with studies indicating that testosterone replacement therapy increases muscle mass and improves grip strength (14). Low bone density is also a characteristic feature of low testosterone levels. Testosterone supplementation significantly improves bone density, stimulates new bone deposition and encourages the laying down of healthy minerals in ailing bones. One 74-year-old gentleman with a history of lower back pain and progressive loss of height, had fortnightly testosterone injections to enhance diminishing levels of this hormone. He soon found that his back had improved and his relationship with his wife received an added boost.

2. TESTOSTERONE AND SEXUAL FUNCTION

Testosterone is essential for sexual desire and libido. When testosterone levels become very low, sex drive becomes virtually non-existent, ejaculation decreases and a sense of depression sets in. UCLA endocrinologists have found that when testosterone is administered to older men their mood improves, libido is renewed and their level of energy increases (15). Whether testosterone alleviates impotence remains a matter of debate. Some men with low testosterone have impotence and benefit from low testosterone supplementation, whereas other men with low testosterone have no problems getting an erection. In the following chapter you will learn more about testosterone's role in promoting sexual vitality.

3. TESTOSTERONE AND THE CARDIOVASCULAR SYSTEM

You've already discovered how important testosterone is for cardiovascular health. Located on the heart muscle are a number of receptors for testosterone. Without it, the heart muscle ceases to pump efficiently. Testosterone stimulates the formation of a substance called nitric oxide synthetase, which is responsible for the formation of nitric oxide. In women, oestrogen generates this chemical, and lo and behold in men, testosterone does exactly the same thing. Nitric oxide is a very potent dilator of blood vessels, so the key to keeping the blood flowing around the body is for each sex to have adequate levels of their own hormones.

Testosterone is now considered such a powerful anti-ischaemic agent that some centres are contemplating using it in the form of intravenous therapy for male heart attack victims who are testosterone deficient.

4. TESTOSTERONE AND WEIGHT LOSS

Populations that live the longest have the best lean body mass. In other words, to live a long and healthy life you have to have more muscle and less fat. If you look around you, you will notice that older men are generally not lean and svelte. As testosterone declines, so does lean body mass. As your lean body mass declines you will find it harder to burn off those extra kilos and you will start to accumulate more body fat. One of the consequences of excess body fat is the development of insulin resistance, which leads to more weight gain and so on and so on. What doctors in the US are now doing is treating insulin resistance with testosterone. They have found that the way to beat this metabolic problem is with testosterone, which is the same route that doctors have taken in treating insulin resistance in women with oestrogen. It's fascinating how symmetrical the biological puzzles of ageing are turning out to be. To circumvent a lot of the difficulties of ageing, especially around heart disease, weight gain and insulin resistance, both sexes simply need to have a good supply of their own hormones.

5. TESTOSTERONE AND THE PROSTATE

Experts are now beginning to agree that testosterone is not the cause of prostate cancer. Insufficient testosterone and the accumulation of oestrogen are the real problems. Testosterone is now being used as a treatment for the enlargement of the prostate, and therapies are also targeting the excessive build-up of oestrogen. Once these imbalances are corrected, the prostate will shrink and the symptoms of prostatic enlargement will diminish.

Measuring Testosterone

Any male who has the typical features of andropause should have their testosterone levels measured. When you do this, make sure that your doctor checks your free testosterone levels either by means of a blood test, or, even better, by means of a salivary hormone sample. For those who need testosterone replacement, natural testosterone is now available in the form of a cream that is synthesised from wild yam. These creams are obtainable from compounding pharmacies located around Australia.

Enhancing Testosterone Naturally

Regular exercise is a must if you want to maintain youthful levels of testosterone. It also prevents weight gain, which is counterproductive to hormonal health. Zinc is important for testosterone production. The herbs tribulus terrestris and Siberian ginseng are testosterone boosters, but we will explore this further when we deal with sexual health in the next chapter.

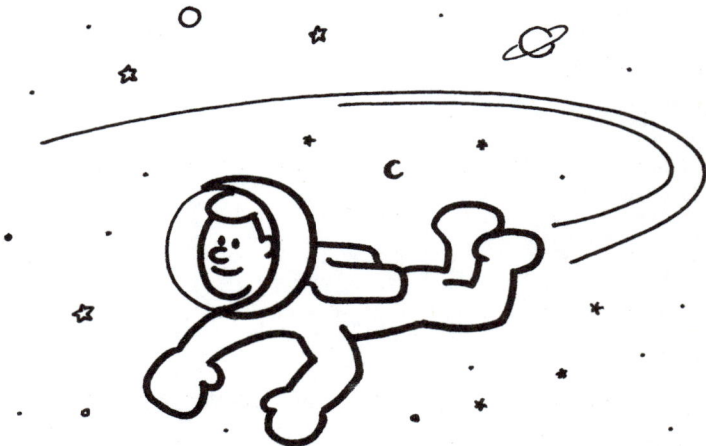

Men rotate in different orbits

Neither sex can live without hormones. For women, the dilemma surrounds the path that is taken to preserve the effects of youthful hormonal levels. For men, maintaining normal hormone levels is equally essential for health and wellbeing.

Key Points To Remember

Oestrogen, progesterone and testosterone play an important part in:

- Promoting cardiovascular health
- Building strong bones
- Preventing the degenerative diseases of ageing
- Maintaining sexual vitality
- Safeguarding the wellbeing of the genito-urinary system

The menopausal transition highlights the difficulties women have in making choices that best promote their health.

Optimal Sexual Vitality

Optimal Sexual Vitality

*T*HE SUPREME EXPRESSION OF ETERNAL HEALTH IS ONGOING sexual vitality. I don't think that anyone would dispute that having a fulfilling sex life is one of nature's most cherished and enjoyable gifts. Woody Allen was once noted to have remarked that his wife used to acknowledge his sexual prowess with a standing ovation, to which George Burns, the ageless American comedian, replied that his audience used to give him a standing ovation simply for standing. Yes, sex is a lot of fun and it is also the healthy embodiment of all our anti-ageing hormones acting in perfect unison. There is so much information, guidance and sexual stimulation out there that you would think that for most of us, having a satisfying sex life would be a mere formality.

Statistics tell us otherwise. With erectile dysfunction reaching epidemic proportions we know that men aren't exactly setting the rafters alight. Women, however, don't appear to be faring any better. In a survey performed in 1994, figures revealed that one

third of American women have entirely lost their interest in sex
(1). When you reflect on all the gains supposedly achieved by
sexual liberation and the notion that uninhibited sexual expression
is every individual's birthright, then these findings are truly
remarkable. If what you see in the movies is any reflection of the
current sexual climate, you'd think that we are all as athletic in
the bedroom as we are on the gym floor. The reality is that we
seem to have lost our way in the intricate dance of intimacy and
sexuality, and for many of us, especially the male sex, a saviour
would be as welcome as a hot chocolate on a cold, rainy day.

All of this has made it a perfect time for Viagra to surface
on the sexual horizon. If ever there was a drug whose time had
come, Viagra was it. Suddenly, with the mere popping of a pill,
men with erectile dysfunction could reverse their fortunes
almost instantaneously. If the flesh was willing, certainly the
spirit wasn't weak. Baby-boomers whose sexual stocks had taken
a nose-dive could now anticipate a life of unbridled sexual
passion as long as their bodies were able to last the distance.
Hail Viagra, the ultimate anti-ageing drug. Although for some
men Viagra has been a godsend, it is certainly not the Messiah.
What we are witnessing is not only a revolution in sexual
behaviour, but in the way men are reflecting on their sexual
health. Viagra may be able to restore erectile ability, but it
cannot enhance libido, nor can it renew energy or wellbeing.
Although men want to improve their performance, they also
want the vitality that comes with it. In order to appreciate how
sexual vitality can be rejuvenated we have to understand what
it is that governs male sexual energy.

The Male Experience

Men are driven by testosterone. To a certain extent this is true for women as well, but men have 10 times the amount coursing through their bodies at any given time. Testosterone goes through daily fluctuations, reaching its peak in the early morning, which is why men are often propelled by sexual desire at that time of day. The male brain is pre-wired to react to testosterone, and besides driving libido, this hormone fuels aggression, dominance and sometimes downright hostility. Testosterone can often get the average male into a lot of trouble as he may find himself acting on impulses over which he has very little control. Men are driven by testosterone to want sex and by nature they are promiscuous, if not in deed then at least in thought. It is the biological imperative that makes men want to spread their seed and connect sex with conquest. Men are doers and if they don't have easy access to the language of love they express affection through acts of kindness rather than by whispering sweet nothings into the ears of their loved ones. The average male struggles with emotions, intimacy and fidelity, all the essential ingredients of a good relationship, because it is simply not in his nature to be part of such an arrangement. Studies have even demonstrated that married men with high testosterone levels have difficulty staying committed. They tend to be abusive, have affairs and regularly end up in the divorce courts (2).

While testosterone may get the poor, hapless male into endless turmoil, without this hormone he is a mere shadow of his former self. Deprive a man of testosterone and his libido will collapse, and in some cases so will his sexual potency. When testosterone levels recede, men become irritable, lethargic and depressed. Give a man a testosterone boost and the whole picture changes. There are a number of studies that confirm that men who have low testosterone benefit substantially from testosterone replacement. Men who have been given testosterone treatment demonstrate increased frequency of sexual thoughts and a marked elevation of sexual desire (3). Sexual arousal is not the only factor that experiences a dramatic resurgence. Further evidence indicates that when testosterone patches are applied to men who are low in testosterone, their erections last longer, they occur more frequently and are more rigid (4). Men who take testosterone generally experience renewed feelings of energy, vitality and wellbeing. Zinc increases testosterone production as does vigorous anaerobic exercise such as weight lifting, whereas regular, exhaustive exercise such as marathon running depletes testosterone.

Aside from testosterone governing sexual potency, to perform effectively men need a healthy blood supply, adequate servings of the molecule nitric oxide and successful management of stress. When the male is sexually aroused, the penis rapidly fills with blood, which is delivered via the penile arteries. If this inflow of blood is rapid enough, the veins that allow blood to flow out of the penis will be compressed preventing any venous escape. This is how an erection is sustained. Nitric oxide's role is to dilate the blood vessels so that the flow of blood proceeds without restriction. Diseases like diabetes and atherosclerosis will gum up the blood vessels supplying the penis, which leads to erectile dysfunction.

We know that stress reduces testosterone levels, but consider how it impacts on sexual activity in another fashion. The whole process of erectile function is mediated by the autonomic nervous system. This part of the nervous system governs involuntary acts and it has two components: parasympathetic and sympathetic. It is the parasympathetic component that facilitates erections and it does this in a calm, relaxed manner. The sympathetic nervous system operates in exactly the opposite fashion, mobilising the body during times of emergency. When the parasympathetic is in control, sexual encounters proceed in an unhurried manner with lots of time to enjoy the experience. But if the sympathetic comes to the fore, suddenly things become incredibly rushed. You may desperately want to prolong the sensation, but if the sympathetic wins you will find yourself losing any say in the matter and before you can regain your composure you will have ejaculated. Sex therapists advise that one of the ways to access the parasympathetic side is to take a deep breath when close to ejaculating. This will override sympathetic input and prevent premature ejaculation.

Excessive stress makes it difficult to initiate parasympathetic activity, which may lead to trouble maintaining an erection. Once you have risen to the occasion, anxiety and worry can activate the sympathetic system, resulting in premature ejaculation once again. Remaining in a parasympathetic state is one of the keys to prolonged, enjoyable sex. It's all very well to have the hormones, chemicals and blood supply, but these won't do you much good if you are overwhelmed by a mountain of stress. This is when relaxation, yoga and meditation can be so beneficial.

Growth hormone and DHEA are the other powerful boosters of sexual energy. Thyroid hormone also needs to be in balance for healthy sexual function to prevail. Another hormone that has recently become popular as a promoter of sexual energy is androstenedione. This is a steroid hormone found in meat and in the pollen of the Scotch pine tree. Taking androstenedione raises testosterone levels and the benefits include increased energy, strength and muscle growth. This is what makes it so popular among athletes, as it increases power and endurance along with heightened sexual arousal. It is important that you realise that if your body is producing adequate amounts of testosterone, androstenedione may not generate additional quantities of this hormone. It is therefore advisable for anyone embarking on a course of hormone supplementation to have their hormone levels checked before and during the course of the program. Regular monitoring of the prostate is also mandatory.

The Female Experience

While men have a simple hormonal deal, women have a complex cocktail of hormones. Although we know some of the factors that drive female sexuality, we do not completely understand what it is that ignites women's sexual instincts. Take testosterone for example. Just as it does for men, testosterone is purported to rule female libido. Testosterone increases most women's sexual arousal and frequency of orgasms. Women with high testosterone levels are more sexually active and they tend to have more muscle and less fat. A study performed recently on 30 working women in New York found that those with higher testosterone levels were more success orientated and not the ones who were in long-term relationships. The women with lower testosterone levels were either married or in stable relationships (5).

Testosterone peaks around ovulation and this is the time when sexual desire is expected to intensify. However, one study has shown that for some women, sexual activity is at its lowest when testosterone levels are at their highest (6). Other findings indicate that female sexual interest is most pronounced around the time of menstruation (7). Although testosterone may arouse libido, it does not necessarily translate into action. In his book entitled Hormonal Health, Dr Michael Colgan maintains that testosterone drops significantly around the time of menopause along with the other hormones. It is this decline that he claims leads to diminished libido, energy and vitality. Dr Colgan has found that adding a touch of testosterone during this period improves confidence, vigour and sexual potency (8).

Testosterone is not the only hormone that influences female sexuality. Oestrogen produced in the first part of the cycle gives a woman her sexual allure. When oestrogen floods the brain, lustful thoughts rage through a woman's mind. Oestrogen makes the genitals more sensitive to touch. When oestrogen is at its peak, women tend to feel more sexy and their desire to procreate heightens. This is a time when a woman is biologically impelled to seek the most suitable mate. Regular sexual intercourse increases oestrogen as does the consumption of the phyto-oestrogens found in peas, beans and soy. Sexual abstinence, extreme weight loss and frequent strenuous exercise reduces oestrogen.

Progesterone, on the other hand, tends to have more of an inhibitory effect on sexuality. During the second half of a woman's cycle, sexual desire decreases and a more relaxed emotional state prevails. Sometimes a woman may feel tired and depressed. Dr John Lee, ever in support of the benefits of progesterone, insists that declining levels of this hormone around menopause also impact on libido. He has found that replacement with small doses of progesterone restores sex drive during this period. Whatever the ultimate truth, there is unquestionably an intricate stew of chemicals constantly pushing and prodding a woman's moods, drives and actions.

Because of this heady mix and the sophisticated wiring system that exists in a woman's brain, the female response to sex is vastly different from the male response. Men are excited by visual stimulation, whereas women prefer to make love in the dark so they can be turned on by the other senses, including taste, smell and touch. Women are better equipped in the auditory department than men which means that the way to a woman's heart is through her ears. Women find it easier to share their feelings because their emotional centre is more closely related to their language centre. If men appear clumsy when articulating their feelings, it's because these two areas are divorced from each other in the male brain. Women desire intimacy and long-term relationships, something that most men have a lot of difficulty coming to terms with. Men are by nature more promiscuous and are impassioned by sexual novelty and athleticism. This does not mean that men are incapable of settling down in a relationship. It merely reaffirms that for the average male, the proverbial sowing of wild oats would probably make it far easier for them to accept a long-term commitment. Recognising and accepting these differences will make it possible for both sexes to get along. If biology is destiny then resisting nature's contribution can consume more energy than it is worth. With waning sexual vitality becoming a feature of everyday life, it appears that both sexes need all the energy they can get. Let's turn our attention now to some of the other means for enhancing sexual vitality.

The Nutrients

When men take Viagra they are increasing the level of a very potent molecule called nitric oxide. You may recall that the role of nitric oxide (NO) is to dilate the blood vessels leading to the penis, which allows for the inflow of blood. Scientists have discovered that taking Viagra is not the only way to raise levels of NO. This can be achieved naturally by means of the amino acid L-arginine.

The scientific community became aware of the benefits of L-arginine in the early 1980s when it was discovered that

L-arginine could stimulate the release of HGH (growth hormone). This coincided with all the wonderful advantages that HGH was found to confer, including boosting sexual vitality. At the end of the 1980s, L-arginine was demonstrated to improve immune function and speed wound healing. Then at the beginning of the 1990s, NO was discovered and the connection between L-arginine, NO and the dilation of blood vessels became apparent.

Since that time, studies have revealed that L-arginine, through the NO connection, offers a powerful means for treating erectile dysfunction. There is evidence that L-arginine gives men erections that are bigger, harder and more frequent than before. By increasing NO, L-arginine is very effective for men who are suffering from blocked arteries due to athero-sclerosis and hypertension.

L-arginine also increases libido. It has been found to be extremely effective when used by women to boost their sexual vitality. One highly athletic 30-year-old woman reported elatedly to her doctor that L-arginine increased her endurance and staying power to six times a night. No prizes for guessing how this doctor reacted to that kind of information.

L-arginine can be found in peanuts, cashews, almonds, garlic, chicken and chocolate, but unfortunately you have to take rather large doses – 4 to 6g – to achieve the desired effect. The best time to take this is approximately 45 minutes before sex. You will also boost HGH release if you avoid eating protein three hours before and two hours after taking L-arginine.

CHOLINE AND VITAMIN B5

Sexual arousal depends on the relay of chemical messages from the brain to the genitals, and this is achieved by means of the neurotransmitter acetylcholine. This is the very same chemical that has a significant part to play in preventing Alzheimer's disease. In the brain, acetylcholine works hand-in-hand with dopamine, which is the feel good chemical. Maintaining optimal levels of both of these chemicals intensifies sexual pleasure. Acetylcholine is involved in the build-up towards orgasm and it prolongs the duration of orgasm. Not a bad deal. And all you have to do to achieve this is to take choline and vitamin B5 just before sex, along with L-arginine if need be. This will allow you to enjoy the sexual experience for a longer period with more energy.

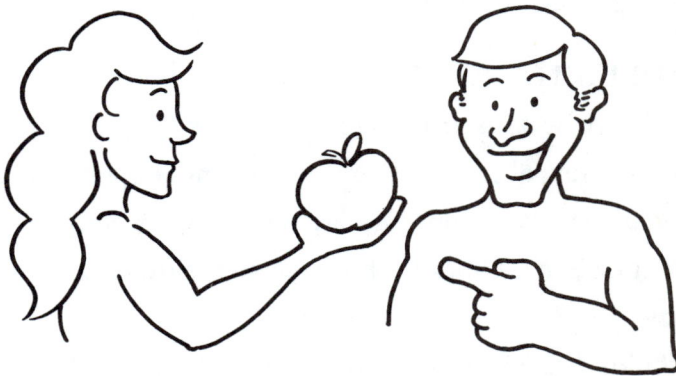

Eve, I wonder if that apple has all those chemicals they keep on talking about

TYROSINE AND PHENYLALANINE

The way to increase dopamine is by taking supplements of the amino acids tyrosine and phenylalanine, together with vitamin B6, vitamin C and folic acid. Chocolate is high in phenylalanine, which may explain why we get a wonderful euphoric feeling every time we indulge ourselves.

The Herbs

Herbal tonics that have been around since the beginning of recorded history have gained popularity as promoters of sexual energy and vitality. The real advantage of herbal treatments is their all-round tonifying effects on a wide range of organ systems. This means that the whole body benefits when you take herbs, and when you throw into the bargain their very low side-effect profile, you have at your disposal the kind of remedy that can only act to your advantage. What are these herbs that have become all the rage for alleviating sexual dysfunction and enhancing sexual pleasure?

TRIBULUS TERRESTRIS

This herb was used in ancient India, where it was found to heighten sexual pleasure. Its rejuvenating properties made it a popular remedy in those times, and it has recently captured the imagination of those who wish to improve their sexual potency.

Tribulus has been noted to enhance libido and it makes erections stronger and last longer. It is also an effective fertility potion as it increases the number and quality of sperm. In women, tribulus boosts sexual energy by promoting ovulation. It also replenishes depleted adrenals, which is important for health and vitality. Symptoms of menopause such as hot flushes, insomnia and irritability can be alleviated with tribulus.

What makes tribulus even more intriguing is its different mechanism of action in men and women. In men it increases testosterone by stimulating the production of luteinising hormone in the pituitary; while in women it boosts the production of follicle-stimulating hormone, which leads to the presence of more oestrogen. Now I know of no drug that has such versatile properties.

Tribulus is an anabolic herb that acts to stimulate muscle growth and improve muscle strength, while enhancing growth hormone production. This makes it a very popular herb with athletes who enjoy the anabolic effects of taking a substance without any negative side-effects.

Individuals who take tribulus also notice diminished lethargy and fatigue, increased mental alertness and tremendous surges of stamina.

DAMIANA

The leaves of this herb were used in America as far back as the 18th century to improve sexual ability. Damiana is currently recognised as an aphrodisiac for both sexes. It is regarded among the natives of Mexico as a stimulant of the sexual apparatus, especially in females. Damiana acts on the central nervous system to overcome exhaustion and help restore hormonal balance. This herb boosts circulation and increases sensitivity to touch in the genital organs. Damiana is alleged to induce erotic fantasies, thereby making the body ready for sexual passion.

GINKGO BILOBA

Ginkgo has already been acknowledged for its brain-stimulating effects due to the fact that it dilates blood vessels. Research work has revealed that ginkgo works just as well in restoring blood to the penis. In a study performed in Germany, 60 men with erectile dysfunction (thought to be caused by poor blood supply) took ginkgo for an extended period of time. After six to eight weeks improvements were noted, and within six months half of the men had regained erectile function (9).

PANAX GINSENG

Ginseng is well known for its ability to revitalise and energise. Those taking ginseng experience renewed energy and markedly diminished levels of fatigue. Ginseng reduces sexual dysfunction by increasing libido and raising testosterone levels.

OATS

This nutrient has been shown to enhance sexual vitality and performance. In a study conducted by the Institute of Human Sexuality in San Francisco, 100 men were given oats over a four-week period followed by four weeks of placebo. Those taking the herb experienced firmer erections, but this effect diminished when they took the placebo. The oldest participants experienced the greatest benefits, enjoying greater sexual desire and overall sexual satisfaction with firmer erections than they had sustained in years. Laboratory tests also found that testosterone levels were increased (10).

In another study, women, too, experienced enhanced sexual desire, performance and genital sensation after taking oats.

NETTLES

Nettles root contains a high concentration of vitamin C, which assists testosterone production, giving the body a natural hormone boost.

MUIRA PUAMA

In South American folklore, this herb is considered to be an aphrodisiac and a treatment for impotence. A study conducted at the Institute of Sexology in Paris, France, performed on 262 men complaining of a lack of sexual desire and inability to attain or maintain an erection, revealed that within two weeks, 62 per cent of the men with low libido reported an increase in their sexual desire and 51 per cent of the men with erectile dysfunction reported improvement (11).

SAW PALMETTO

This herb is well known for its beneficial effects on the prostate. It also benefits both sexes with regard to improving sexual potency.

All of these herbs can be taken in combination. They make for a powerful array of rejuvenating tonics that enhance sexual energy and youthful vitality.

Exercising For Good Sex

Sexual health is inseparable from overall health. It's really a two-way street. If your sex life is good then your health will benefit and vice versa. One sure way to guarantee a good sex life, all other factors being accounted for, is to have regular exercise. If you are fit and healthy then you are more likely to be able to get up to all sorts of delightful acrobatics in the bedroom.

There have been a host of studies to substantiate these claims. There is no doubt about it: regular exercise leads to regular sex. If you really want to become a sexual athlete, then what you have to do is enrol in a workout program that involves a combination of weight training and aerobic exercise such as jogging. Subjects who were involved in such a study noticed that over a nine-month period they had sex more often and their orgasms were more frequent and satisfying (12). In other words the fitter you are the better the sex. Moderate exercise on the treadmill three to four times a week certainly is a start, but if you want to be an iron man or woman in between the sheets then you have to step up your exercise regimen. Do this gradually and enjoy it. Remember, like sex, exercise should be a lot of fun.

When you exercise regularly you increase your levels of HGH and testosterone, which have all those beneficial effects on your body, while enhancing your sex drive at the same time. What a bargain! A regular workout promotes blood flow to all parts of your body and builds cardiovascular efficiency. When you consider that one of the major causes of impotence is arterial blockage, keeping your blood vessels patent and pliable through frequent exercise is essential.

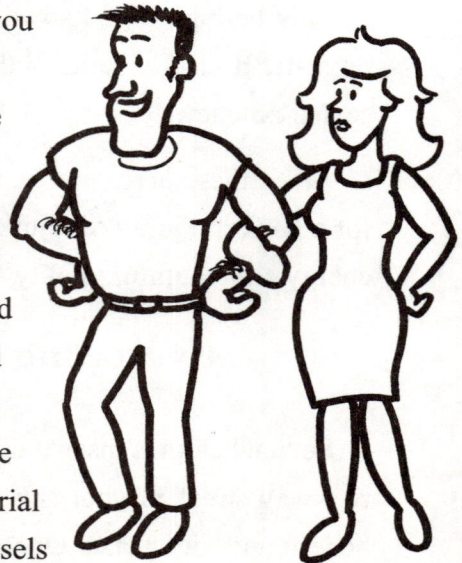

Hmmm, I wonder if he really is a sexual athlete

Key Points To Remember

In men, sexual vitality depends on:

- Testosterone
- HGH
- DHEA

In women, sexual vitality depends upon a complex interplay of the following:

- Oestrogen
- Progesterone
- Testosterone
- DHEA

Nutrients and herbs that boost sexuality include:

- L-arginine
- Choline
- Vitamin B5
- Tyrosine
- Phenylalanine
- Tribulus Terrestris
- Damiana
- Ginkgo Biloba
- Panax Ginseng
- Oats
- Nettles
- Muira Puama
- Saw Palmetto

Fighting Obesity
And Fatigue

Fighting Obesity And Fatigue

*I*F YOU ARE OVERWEIGHT AND DON'T HAVE ENOUGH ENERGY TO negotiate your average day, then you are manifesting the early warning signs of premature ageing. These are the cardinal signs that your anti-ageing hormones are out of sync and your body has gone into reverse gear. What you need to do is find out how you can turn this whole process around so that you feel renewed and revitalised. This will mean that you have restored your body's metabolic process to its youthful efficiency and that your anti-ageing hormones are doing exactly what they do best—keeping you young and vital. You have to realise that this is no easy task. Current trends indicate that if you want to differentiate yourself from the pack, then you have to make a concerted effort. Statistics show that for the average individual, being overweight and lethargic is a sad fact of everyday life. Tragically, we appear to be less healthy than we ever have been.

One thing is for sure, we are a fatter society than any other in the history of Western civilisation. Some experts estimate that close to a staggering 50 per cent of adult Americans are overweight, and there is every indication that the adult population of Australia isn't far behind. The truth is that the older we get, the fatter we become, and the fatter we become the more we place ourselves at risk of getting a serious disease. Once you start to put on weight you increase your risk of succumbing to a number of killer diseases such as diabetes, stroke, heart disease and cancer. If you want to avoid this kind of health disaster then you have to understand the factors that contribute to weight gain, or, more specifically, fat enhancement, as you age.

For those of you who think that you only have to start worrying about being overweight when you finally arrive at middle age, think again. Premature ageing commences in childhood when the tendency to obesity is initiated. This is the bold claim of Dr Henry Anhalt, the Director of Paediatric Endocrinology at the Maimonedes Medical Centre, Brooklyn, New York (1). Dr Anhalt reveals that overweight statistics do not apply to adults alone. Nearly half of all American children are overweight, with over 30 per cent falling into the category of obese. Although Australian children are not faring as badly, trends show that obesity levels in this country have increased over the past two decades. What Dr Anhalt is at pains to point out is that childhood obesity leads to adult obesity. This probability escalates with increasing age along the following lines. An overweight infant has a 14 per cent chance of being an overweight adult, and this figure rises to 41 per cent at age seven, 75 per cent at age 12 and a colossal 90 per cent at adolescence. This is a strong indication that trends are established at a very early age and that if we are going to make meaningful inroads on this metabolic death-sentence then the time to intervene is in childhood.

I'm pleased I can finally fit into these skinny genes

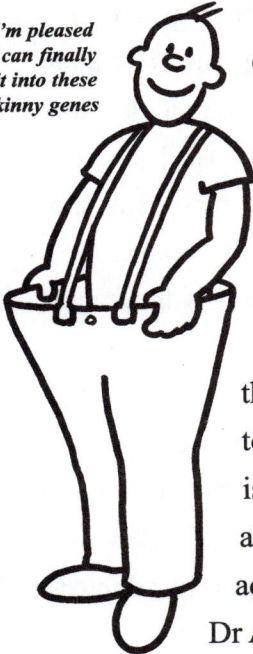

What happens is that you are born with a certain amount of fat cells that get bigger if your eating habits result in weight gain. Not only do your fat cells become larger, but you also begin to make more fat cells. These cells remain with you as you approach adulthood and they become rather difficult to shed. This means that we have to prevent weight gain in the form of fat during this early period. The time to be tough and to initiate weight-loss programs is during childhood when it is easier to bring about metabolic changes, rather than during adulthood when it becomes an uphill struggle.

Dr Anhalt reminds us that our society is less active than it used to be. Not long ago we were hunting on the plains. We had to make a fire by rubbing two sticks together and we had to defend our homes and families against all sorts of wild and vicious animals. All this involved quite an expenditure of energy, and it was entirely appropriate that after such a hard day at the office we enjoyed a hefty meal at the dinner table. These days many of us spend most of our working hours in a sedentary position, then we drive to the supermarket, park as close as we can to the entrance, grab some frozen dinner off the shelf and drive home where we nuke our food in the microwave. We also tend to consume way in excess of our energy expenditure.

Children have adopted similar patterns of behaviour. They spend countless hours in front of the television set or the computer while they munch away on all sorts of fat-promoting snack foods. Obese children have high blood pressure, which begins at a very early age, and they have a propensity to develop lower back pain and arthritis. Obese young girls tend to over-produce male sex hormones, which leads to hirsutism and abnormal periods—as if being overweight isn't enough of a curse! Both sexes have insulin resistance, which is the major precursor to a host of metabolic disorders.

So what does Dr Anhalt propose? He suggests that the whole family should be involved in the treatment program. It's pointless for parents to send their children to therapy when they are setting a bad example. Realistic eating and behaviour goals have to be established, to which everybody adheres. He also emphasises that treatment is a lifelong undertaking and that patterns of eating, exercise and behaviour have to be maintained forever.

If starting off on the wrong foot makes it tough to lose weight, what is it about increasing age that makes it so difficult to shed those extra kilos? Hormonal changes are the major culprits that promote weight gain as we get older.

We already know that HGH and DHEA are centrally located in this issue. As we get older, fat increases while muscle tissue decreases. This coincides with the decline in HGH and DHEA production, which stimulates muscle production while reducing fat. Thyroid hormone also undergoes gradual decline, leading to reduced metabolic rate and weight gain. Because there is less HGH, less DHEA, less thyroid hormone and reduced muscle tissue, we burn less calories from the food we eat than when we were younger. What this translates into is the necessity to reduce food consumption as we get older, or alternatively, exercise a whole lot more if we don't want to put on weight.

The other villain in this story is that old arch-enemy of weight loss—insulin. This is the hormone that opens the door to your cells so that glucose can enter where it is used for energy. When you gain weight your cells become resistant to the effects of insulin. As a consequence, you don't burn glucose very efficiently, nor do you utilise your fat resources for energy purposes. Your body becomes a novice at using glucose effectively and an expert at storing fat. To complete this sad and sorry metabolic tale, obesity decreases HGH and DHEA production, making it even more difficult to lose weight. Gaining fat around the midriff, which happens so often in this type of situation, is of particular concern because central obesity is associated with heart disease, increased incidence of strokes, and can lead to various cancers such as those of the breast, uterus and possibly the ovary.

To reverse this metabolic nightmare you need to adopt certain patterns of behaviour, some of which you will have to maintain for the rest of your life. Diets that are high in bread, rice, potato and cereal, which are alluded to earlier in this book, lead to insulin resistance. This is further exacerbated by a high-fat diet. What you need to do is to consume more plant-based foods that provide you with the necessary ratios of proteins, carbohydrates and fats to keep your insulin levels down and your weight optimal. These include spinach, broccoli, eggplant, legumes, apples, peaches, lentils, soybean curd, almonds, cashews and avocados. If you are still battling to deal with excess insulin, taking supplements of the minerals chromium and zinc will help you to beat this recalcitrant hormone. Doing all you can to boost your production of HGH and DHEA will also counteract the effects of insulin. Naturally, exercise will help you in your endeavours, providing you follow all the principles that I have outlined.

Animal studies demonstrate that food restriction leads to a longer lifespan. Although this may be a hard ask, if you eat sensibly and reduce your food intake to that which keeps you energised and healthy, you may not find it that difficult to maintain your optimal weight.

Fatigue

Excessive fatigue is the other sign that you are in metabolic decline. If you struggle to get out of bed in the morning, your zip and zap has manifestly fizzled, and your boundless energy has dwindled to an alarming crawl, then your body is screaming at you to pay attention. This is a clear indication that your metabolic processes are not proceeding as they should, and if you don't do something about it immediately, you could be staring down the barrel of something akin to chronic fatigue syndrome. Lethargy and diminishing energy are considered to be the beacons of premature ageing. These symptoms are telling you that a host of unfavourable events are taking place in your body and these may include all or some of the following:

• Your anti-ageing hormones are in decline

• Your mitochondria are not generating enough energy to sustain you

• Your digestive process is not providing you with the vital nutrients you need

• Your liver is not eliminating toxins from your body efficiently

In order to discover exactly which system is malfunctioning, you need to undergo the appropriate tests, and in the next chapter you will discover what these are. When it comes to treatment, however, hormones still seem to hold all the aces.

Consider the following circumstance. You awake in the morning and your body is craving a sugar hit. So you go to the refrigerator and you wolf down a sizeable slice of last night's cheesecake followed by a piece of toast with jam and a cup of coffee with sugar. This culinary feast sends an express wake-up call to your pancreas, which releases a substantial salvo of insulin to cope with the sugar load. Excessive insulin causes your blood sugar to drop too low, creating a kind of alarm or stress state in your body. As a result, you need another dose of sugar. This brings the adrenals—the major stress-fighting glands—into play with a huge flourish. The hormone cortisol, that old nemesis, ensures that enough sugar becomes available, which causes another huge upswing in insulin, and you get caught in a destructive metabolic cycle that leads to the premature ageing of your body.

Adrenals that are overworked eventually become exhausted, and this is when fatigue sets in. Constant stress leads to a steady stream of cortisol, which ultimately weakens your muscles, bones and immune system. This is what makes cortisol the ageing hormone and places the adrenal glands firmly in the centre of the anti-ageing saga. Remember that when your adrenals are focused on producing cortisol, DHEA—the other major adrenal hormone—will be compromised. DHEA, as you may recall, does the opposite of cortisol. When your adrenals are not overtaxed and your levels of DHEA and cortisol are in harmony with each other, then you will experience feelings of energy and wellbeing, your sexual vitality will be renewed, and your emotional state will be calm and tranquil.

In reality, how many of us attain this type of daily functioning? Most of us are constantly stressed, producing way too much cortisol and not nearly enough DHEA. Our adrenal glands are triggered by persistent anger, worry and fear. Overwork, insufficient sleep, binge eating and repeated illness place unremitting demands on our resources, which ultimately leads to adrenal exhaustion.

If you experience excessive fatigue, weakness, irritability, cravings for sweet foods and insomnia then your adrenals are run down and you need to make some timely changes. This is an ideal time to revisit the second chapter in order to refresh your memory about DHEA renewal.

Relaxing regularly with a meditation tape, listening to music that you love and performing a deep breathing exercise for a few moments each day will reduce some of the damaging effects of stress on your adrenals. Dealing with emotional conflict will send a very powerful message to your adrenals that your life is under control and that there is no need to mobilise for 'fight or flight'. If you look after your adrenals then you will allow cortisol—the ageing hormone—to take a back seat, and DHEA—the hormone of youth and vitality—to come to the fore.

Needless to say, the other anti-ageing hormones are also primarily involved in generating energy. HGH and thyroid hormone need to be maintained at optimal levels to sustain youthful vitality. Hence the massive drive to find ways to preserve youthful levels of HGH in anti-ageing centres around the globe.

The other two principle players in the fatigue equation are the gut and the liver. We need the digestion process to be functioning adequately to provide all the vital nutrients that are the building blocks for our anti-ageing hormones. Once the gut has fulfilled its obligations, it's up to the liver to deal effectively with all the toxins that have accumulated in the body so that they can be eliminated. If the liver fails to do its job, toxins will establish themselves in the guise of free-radicals, and their first port of call will be the poor mitochondria. Mitochondrial DNA that has been damaged is not able to replicate very successfully, if at all. Without enough mitochondria, cells become starved of energy and eventually cell death occurs. Organs then cease to function effectively and this loss of organ reserve is what ageing is all about.

Fatigue is a very common symptom of modern-day living and it is also one of the early indications of premature ageing.

If dealt with promptly, adverse metabolic events can be prevented before they cause any enduring disasters.

Key Points To Remember

Obesity is caused by:
• Childhood patterns of behaviour and eating
• Sedentary lifestyle
• Insufficient exercise
• Insulin resistance
• The decline in HGH, DHEA and thyroid hormone

Fatigue is related to:
• Low levels of anti-ageing hormones
• Excessive cortisol stimulation
• Mitochondrial burn-out
• Poor digestion
• Inadequate liver detoxification

Diet, Lifestyle And The Biomarkers Of Ageing

Diet, Lifestyle And
The Biomarkers
Of Ageing

I DON'T KNOW ABOUT YOU, BUT I HAVEN'T COME ACROSS MANY folk who are overflowing with energy. I would actually say that the opposite is true. My average working day is chock-full of patients who suffer from a lack of energy and vitality, poor mental function, bad digestive systems, diminished libidos and recurrent bouts of illness. In other words, these folk are displaying all the signs of accelerated ageing. These are the unfortunate individuals who have run the gamut of standard medical testing only to be told that there is nothing wrong with them. At least nothing that these tests can uncover. This is where medicine, as we currently experience it, is failing us. Even today, medical practice addresses illness and not wellness. But what most of us need to know is: what is it that is going wrong in our bodies to make us unhealthy? We need to know about the metabolic imbalances that prevent us from experiencing real vitality. Most importantly, we need to know how to maintain a healthy internal biochemical environment. This is what makes the science of anti-ageing medicine so timely.

New technologies have been developed that allow us to identify the exact biochemical factors that lead to all the features of accelerated ageing. Long before your body succumbs to the degenerative diseases of ageing you can be aware of the reasons why you are losing your youthful vitality. This will allow you to replace symptoms of ill-health with robust wellness for as long as you desire. Everyone has the right to Eternal Health, and it is possible for you to continue to enjoy your life with childlike enthusiasm and vigour. There are cultures where this very achievement is a fact of everyday life. The old folk survive to a ripe old age, free of the degenerative diseases so characteristic of Western civilisation.

Lifestyle

In cultures such as the Vilcabambans from the Andes of Ecuador, the Bilcabambans of Peru, and the Abkhasians who live on the eastern shores of the Black Sea it is not uncommon to find elders who live to the ripe old age of 120, and they don't expect a telegram from the Queen honouring their achievement.

The whole ethic around ageing is quite different in these cultures. The elderly remain active well into their latter years and it is expected of them. This is especially true of sexual activity, with many of the these elderly folk sustaining active sex lives well beyond the age of 100, a feat virtually unheard of in our culture.

These societies have very little stress and their lives don't revolve around deadlines or the pressures of time. As they often don't have electricity, their daily patterns are determined by the rhythms of nature. They rise with the sun and go to sleep when it sets. Resting is considered of prime importance and they enjoy long siestas and spend more time sleeping at night. This allows HGH to kick in.

The diets of these communities is mostly vegetarian. They consume a variety of greens and vegetables including cauli-flower, cabbage, broccoli and zucchini. Fruit trees rich with mangoes, berries, cherries and bananas are plentiful. Most importantly, they eat their fruit and vegetables raw, a factor that seems to contribute to their good digestive systems.

Another element that contributes to the longevity of these societies is the richness of their soil and water. Their water comes from natural springs and contains an abundant supply of minerals including calcium, zinc, selenium and magnesium. Their fields are heavily laden with carbon and phosphorus as well as other essential nutrients. Hair mineral analyses performed on these people confirm that they have an abundance of protective nutrients. Heavy metal toxins such as lead, mercury and aluminium are nowhere to be found. Degenerative diseases are virtually unheard of. Arthritis, heart disease and cancer are practically extinct. Not surprisingly, these villages are filled with folk who engage in daily activities with the laughter and merriment normally associated with small children. It is no wonder that they live to a ripe old age, free of illness and full of boundless vitality.

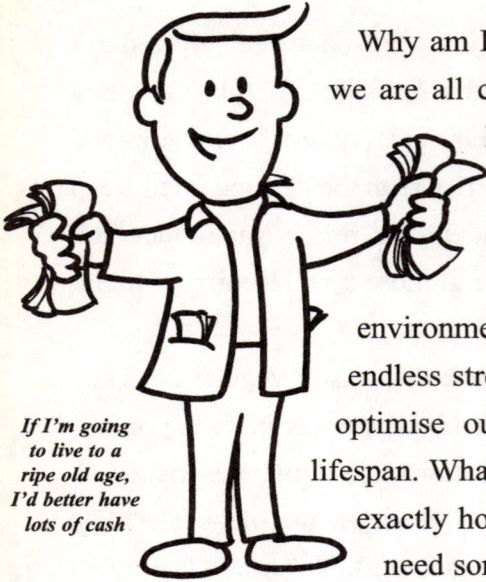

If I'm going to live to a ripe old age, I'd better have lots of cash

Why am I telling you all this? Because we are all capable of enjoying the same healthy journey into longevity that is achieved in these cultures. Even though we are subject to a much harsher environment full of toxic pollutants and endless stresses and strains, we can still optimise our health and maximise our lifespan. What we need to do is to find out exactly how healthy our bodies are. We need some form of objective measure that will tell us how successfully we are negotiating the ageing process. This is what the biomarkers of ageing are all about. These are the tests that evaluate the biological and biochemical status of your body. Your biomarkers will inform you whether you are in line to develop any of the dreaded diseases of ageing, and will give you pointers as to how you can avoid them. You will discover ways of improving your health and restoring the vitality that is missing in your life. That is if your experience is similar to that which I encounter in my daily practice. These are the tests that will supersede the current batch of medical investigations. This is what 21st century medicine will be all about. The biomarkers of ageing, which are all about evaluating health and wellbeing rather than ill-health and disease, will usher in a totally new paradigm in health care delivery. Welcome to the future.

The Biomarkers Of Ageing

1. THE HORMONAL BIOMARKERS

These comprise all the anti-ageing hormones including HGH, DHEA, melatonin and thyroid hormone, as well as the other hormones mentioned in this book such as cortisol, oestrogen, progesterone and testosterone. HGH, thyroid hormone and testosterone can be measured by means of blood tests, whereas the others should be evaluated by salivary assays. With regard to DHEA and cortisol, it is a good idea to have samples taken twice a day so that you get a true reflection of the daily fluctuations in these hormones. This will also provide you with valuable information as to how your body is dealing with stress. Likewise, melatonin should be sampled in the morning and evening so that you get some idea of the peak and baseline levels. For post-menopausal women, some medical authorities regard oestrogen and progesterone as worthless assays, however, I am of the opinion that these hormones should be maintained within certain parameters so assessing these hormones is useful. Testosterone holds the key to sexual vitality for both sexes so it is a very necessary test.

Once you have a compilation of all your hormones, you then need a program that will restore them to optimal levels. The relevant chapters in this book provide you with the means to do just that. You should have your hormone levels monitored regularly to ensure that you are maintaining appropriate levels. Remember that preserving the right balance is the key.

2. THE BIOLOGICAL TERRAIN ASSESSMENT

The Biological Terrain Assessment (BTA) has become one of the primary tools used in anti-ageing clinics around the world to evaluate the internal biochemical environment of the body. The term terrain is used because the noted professor who devised this test, Louis Claude Vincent, viewed the body as a garden, which, if filled with soil that is well tendered and rich with nutrients and minerals, will yield a good seed. Similarly, our biological garden is the chemistry of our body that needs to be in balance if good health is to ensue. Professor Vincent believed that by focusing on the uniqueness of each individual's biochemistry, he could discover the secrets that lead to optimal health. Specifically, he targeted the bodily fluids, saliva, urine and blood, and what he did was to measure three different parameters: pH, redox and resistivity. He considered these to embrace the essence of body biochemistry and he was able to gather data that helped identify imbalances and problem areas. He was then able to suggest the appropriate changes thereby re-establishing health and vitality in previously sick patients. These tests are now used to provide the earliest indication of accelerated ageing and they are speedily becoming the gold standard for anti-ageing assessments. Interestingly, a lot of patients who report normal blood tests display abnormal results on the BTA, indicating that they have biochemical abnormalities that aren't being identified by standard medical tests. These are the individuals who suffer from fatigue, poor digestion, impaired memory and all the other symptoms mentioned earlier, which need to be addressed before any long-term damage sets in.

The BTA is just the test they need to set them on the right track. Let's take a closer look at the parameters developed to isolate biochemical abnormalities, namely pH, redox and resistivity.

pH

This is a measure of the degree of acidity and alkalinity in the various bodily fluids. The body constantly attempts to maintain the pH within the optimal range. However, if our diets are high in animal protein and simple sugars and we have lots of stress, then we tend to produce acids that may disrupt cellular metabolism and interfere with enzyme systems, creating the potential for diseases to develop and premature ageing. Once acids accumulate, it's up to the liver and kidneys to eliminate these from the body. A BTA test will tell you whether the pH of your urine, saliva and blood are too acid or too alkaline, and from this you'll be able to gauge whether you have the right diet and whether your kidneys, liver and digestive system are carrying out their proper functions. If not, you can make the appropriate adjustments to rectify the situation.

REDOX

This is probably the most important component of the BTA assessment as it tells you how well your body is coping with free-radicals and whether your antioxidant defences are adequate. Specifically, you will discover how your mitochondria are holding up against the ever-increasing free-radical menace, as they are most vulnerable to attack by these substances. If your redox values are too high, you may need to take supplementary antioxidants.

RESISTIVITY

This component of the BTA assessment tells you about your mineral status. When mineral concentrations are too low, which is commonly seen in osteoporosis, resistivity goes up. Conversely, when your mineral levels are too high, this usually indicates a buildup of mineral salts, which is a reflection of inadequate lymphatic drainage and kidney elimination.

These tests provide you with vital information as to how your body is performing those chemical and biological reactions essential to health and life. By carrying out the BTA assessment, you will discover whether you are digesting and eliminating efficiently, and whether you are dealing effectively with the toxins accumulating in your body. The BTA pinpoints weaknesses and imbalances and tells you how to go about correcting them so that you can restore your terrain to its best function.

3. GUT AND LIVER BIOMARKERS

Once you have completed the BTA assessment you will have some idea as to whether you are absorbing the nutrients from which anti-ageing hormones and other key substances are manufactured. If you have persistent gut symptoms, then you may need to take the tests referred to in Chapter 3 such as the CDSA and the intestinal permeability test. The liver is an equally important player in the anti-ageing process as not only does it purge our body of toxins, but it modulates essential anti-ageing hormones such as HGH and thyroid hormone, which only become active after they have been transformed by the liver. If you have signs of persistent liver dysfunction such as dry scalp, easy bruising and constant exhaustion, in addition to the BTA, you may have to take a test that assesses the functional capabilities of your liver. This is different from a standard blood test, and ARL laboratory in Melbourne can provide you with the necessary information regarding this test (address at the back of the book).

4. MENTAL BIOMARKERS

Diseases such as Alzheimer's and Parkinson's disease develop slowly and progressively. By performing tests that assess memory, reaction time, visual and auditory capability, together with an evaluation of the levels of the essential neurotransmitters acetylcholine, serotonin and dopamine, mental decline can be detected long before symptoms develop and the disease process sets in. This will allow you to avert any of these neurodegenerative diseases before they set up shop in your body.

5. CARDIOVASCULAR BIOMARKERS

Aside from the established risk factors for heart disease, you now have to ensure that your levels of homocysteine, lipoprotein(a) and fibrinogen are kept to a minimum. This can be achieved with vitamins B6, B12, folic acid, vitamin C and the amino acid lysine. Measuring these new parameters will soon become a standard component of any comprehensive cardiovascular assessment.

6. BODY COMPOSITION

With ageing, muscle mass decreases and fat accumulates, increasing the risk of heart disease, diabetes and stroke. The relative distribution of fat and muscle around your body is a reflection of your hormones in action and will also impact on the function of your hormones. Maintaining good muscle mass will assist you in preserving HGH levels and will promote good cardiovascular health. A bioelectrical impedance analysis is the new technology that has been developed to accurately assess the muscle and fat percentages in your body.

7. BONE DENSITY

A lack of exercise, a decline in oestrogen, testosterone, progesterone and the anti-ageing hormones, combined with a diet deficient in the essential minerals calcium and magnesium, contributes to the demineralisation of your bones. This process commences before menopause and its effect on men is grossly underestimated. This is why it is important to look after your bones from a very early age and to have your bone density checked regularly as you get older.

8. IMMUNE BIOMARKERS

The potency of your immune system diminishes with age as you find yourself increasingly at the mercy of internal and external invaders. Your T-cells are responsible for adjusting your immune response to impending threat. T-helper cells activate the other components of the immune system, whereas T-suppressor cells prevent the overproduction of anti-bodies. It is important to preserve the normal ratio of T-helper to T-suppressor cells as you age otherwise you run the risk of developing auto-immune diseases such as rheumatoid arthritis.

Having completed your biomarker assessment, you will have an intimate view of the biochemical workings of your body, and you will find out what it is that is holding you back from ideal health. Once you have optimised your biomarker status you will be well on the road to vitality and longevity. All that remains is for you to sort out the best possible diet for your unique biochemistry.

The Diet

Although I do endorse individuality as far as diets are concerned, as a general rule I am pro-vegetarian. Besides the environmental and humanitarian perspective, if we want to emulate the achievements of the long-lived populations of the world it looks like vegetarianism is the way to go. It works for them and so why shouldn't it work for us?

What I tell my patients to do is to consume fruits and vegetables in abundance. These need to be in season and should be eaten raw as often as possible. This type of dietary practice has a number of advantages. Fruit and vegetables are considered alkaline-producing foods as opposed to acid-forming foods like dairy products, animal based proteins and cereal grains. An alkaline environment is much more favourable to the activities of our hormones and enzyme systems. Fruits and vegetables are also rich in natural antioxidants that protect us against the number one promoter of ageing—the proliferation of free-radicals.

In addition to fruit and vegetables, if we consume a healthy supply of nuts and seeds we will provide further support for the various organ systems of our body. The really important question then is: will diet alone be enough to provide you with all the nutrients you need to promote world-beating health? If you've completed your biomarker assessment you will realise that some form of nutrient supplementation is absolutely essential. Even if you have the best vegetarian diet that nature can provide with organic fruit and vegetables in season, it still won't be possible for you to secure all the antioxidants, vitamins, minerals and amino-acids you need to keep your cells operating in the best possible fashion. Every single one of us needs a supplement program. What form this takes depends primarily on the outcome of your biomarker assessment, and any other investigations that are relevant to your current health status.

In my experience, it is extremely rare to find someone whose biological age is on a par with their chronological age. Precious few individuals display the kind of health and energy that is so characteristic of those cultures mentioned earlier, where centenarians are a dime a dozen. This can change. In fact, it has to change if we want to preserve the diminishing resources of this planet. Eternal Health is not a dream. It can become a reality if we rediscover some of the secrets so obvious to the primitive societies of our world.

Key Points To Remember

The biomarkers of ageing clearly define the biochemical and physiological status of your body. These include:

- The hormonal biomarkers
- The Biological Terrain Assessment
- The gut and liver biomarkers
- The mental biomarkers
- The cardiovascular biomarkers
- The immune biomarkers
- Body composition
- Bone density

If you consume the foods that are appropriate for your unique biochemistry, take the necessary supplements, and optimise your biomarker status, you will be well on the way to Eternal Health.

Bibliography

CHAPTER 1.

1. Harman, D., Free-Radical Theory of Ageing, The Science of Anti-Ageing Medicine, pp15–32, 1996.
2. Klatz, R.M., Live fast, love hard, die young & leave a beautiful memory—No way, say the new young doctors, let's live forever!, 3. Anti-Ageing Medical Therapeutics Vol. 2, pp1–8, 1998.
4. Winter, R.M.S., The Anti-Ageing Hormones, Three Rivers Press, New York, 1997.
5. Yanick, P.Jr. and Giampapa, V.C., Quantum Longevity, Promotion Publishing, San Diego, 1997.
6. Statistics of the National Heart Foundation, Australia, 1999.

Additional Resources
1. Yanick, P., Jr. and Giampapa, V.C., Prohormone Nutrition, Longevity Institute International, New Jersey, 1998.
2. Klatz, R.M., Hormones of Youth, Sports Tech Labs, Inc. 1999.

CHAPTER 2.

1. Skrecky, D., The Cause Of Ageing, North Dakota State University Experiment. Longevity, Report 33, p 4, 1999.
2. Rudman, D. et al., Effects Of Human Growth Hormone in men over 60 years old, New England Journal of Medicine, 323, pp1–6, 1990.
3. Fazio, S., Preliminary Study of Growth Hormone in the treatment of dilated cardiomyopathy, New England Journal of Medicine, 334, pp809–814, 1996.
4. South, J., Growth Hormone, The Real Fountain of Youth, IAS Bulletin Extract, pp1–7, March 1999.
5. Wuster, C., et al., Effects of Growth Hormone in bone metabolism in adults, University of Heidelberg, Germany. Poster exhibit at the American Academy of Anti-Ageing Medicine-Annual Conference, December, 1998.
6. Verhaeghe, J. et al., Effects of combined IGF-1 and 17 Beta-Oestradiol on bone turnover in ovariectomized rats, Academisch Ziekenhuis Utrecht, The Netherlands. Poster exhibit at the American Academy of Anti-Ageing Medicine-Annual Conference, December 1998.
7. Jamieson, J. and Dorman, L. E., The Methulasah Factor, Safegoods, East Canaan, 1997.
8. Kroboth, K. D., et al., DHEA and DHEA-S: A Review, J Clin Pharmacol, 39, pp327–348, 1999.
9. Yen, S.S.C., et al., DHEA and Ageing, Annals of the New York Academy of Sciences, 774, pp128–142, 1995.
10. Labrie, F., et al., DHEA and the intracrine formation of androgens and estrogens in peripheral target tissues: Its role during ageing, Steroids, 63, pp322–328, 1998.
11. Colgan, M., Hormonal Health, Apple Publishing, Vancouver, 1996.
12. Maestroni, G. and Pierpaoli, W., Research work reported in reference 13.
13. Pierpaoli, W., Melatonin, The pineal gland and ageing: A planetary and biological reality, The Science of Anti-Ageing Medicine, pp107–114, 1996.

14. Lissoni, P. et al., Neuroimmunotherapy with subcutaneous low-dose Interleukin-2 and The Pineal Hormone Melatonin, Reported in Hormones of Youth, Klatz, R.M., Sports Tech Labs, Inc, Chicago.

Additional Resources
1. Klatz, R. and Goldman, R., Stopping the Clock, Bantam Books, New York, 1996.
2. Sahelian, R., Melatonin: Nature's Sleeping Pill, Be Happier Press, Marina Del Ray, 1995.
3. Sahelian, R., DHEA: A Practical Guide, Avery Publishing Group, New York, 1996.

CHAPTER 3.

1. Drossman, D.A. et al., Factors related to intestinal permeability, Dig Dis Sci, 38, pp1569–1580, 1993.
2. Walker, M., Bovine Colostrum offers broad spectrum benefits for wide-ranging ailments, Townsend Letter, 189, pp74–80, April 1999.

Additional Resources
1. Bland, J., The 20 Day Rejuvenation Diet Program, Keats Publishing Inc, New Canaan, Connecticut, 1997.
2. Braverman, E.R., The Healing Nutrients Within, Keats Publishing, Inc, New Canaan, 1997.
3. Cabot, S., The Healthy Liver and Bowel Book, WHAS, Cobbity, NSW, 1999.
4. D'Adamo, P., The Eat Right Diet, Century, London, 1998.
5. Golan, R., Optimal Wellness, Ballantine Books, New York, 1995.
6. Howell, E., Food Enzymes for Health and Longevity, Lotus Press, Twin Lakes, Wisconson, 1994.
7. Kaminski, M.V., The Gut/Liver/Free-Radical Connection to Ageing, Anti-Aging Medical Therapeutics, pp183–190, 1997.

CHAPTER 4.

1. Martin, W., Reducing deaths from heart attacks and cancer, Townsend Letter, 174, pp72–76, January 1998.
2. French, R., Healthy Hearts, International Wellbeing, 76, pp34–40, June 1999.
3. Islam, K.N. et al., Alpha-tocopherol enrichment of monocytes decreases agonist-induced adhesion to human endothelial cells, Circulation, 98, pp2255–2261, 1998.
4. Barrett-Connor, E., Sex Differences in Coronary Heart Disease: Why are Women so superior?, Circulation, 95(1), pp252–264, 1997.
5. De Rosa N. et al., Impairment of endothelial functions by acute hyperhomocysteinemia and reversal by antioxidant vitamins, JAMA, 281(22), pp213–218, 1999.
6. Wright, J.V., Testosterone: Hormone of the heart, Townsend Letter, 189, pp56–66, April 1999.
7. Hu, F. B. et al., A prospective study of egg consumption and risk of cardiovascular disease in men and women, JAMA, 281, pp1387–1394, 1999.

Additional Resources
1. West, M., Endothelial Function and Vascular Disease: An Evolving Story, Adis, 1998.
2. Henderson, A., Coronary Heart Disease: Overwiew, The Lancet, 348 (1S), pp1–4, 1996.
3. Koenig, W. et al., C-Reactive Protein, a sensitive marker of inflammation, Circulation, 99(2), pp237–242, 1999.
4. Colquhon, D., The Endothelium, Adis, 1999.
5. Levine, M. et al., Criteria and recommendations for vitamin C intake, JAMA, 281, pp1415–1423, 1999.
6. Scott, C.H. and Sutton, M.S., Homocysteine: Evidence for a causal relationship with cardiovascular disease, Cardiol. Rev., 7 (2), pp101–107, 1999.
7. Danesh, J. et al., Chronic Infections and coronary heart disease: Is there a link?, The Lancet, 350 (9075), pp430–436, 1997.

8. Kwang Kon, K. et al., Vascular effects of oestrogen and cholesterol lowering therapies in hypercholeserolemic postmenopausal women, Circulation, 99 (3), pp354–360, 1999.

9. Libby, P., Atheroma: More than mush, The Lancet, 348(1S), pp4–7, 1996.

10. Kromhout, D., Diet-Heart issues in a pharmacological era, The Lancet, 348 (1S), pp20–22, 1996.

11. Andreotti, F. et al., Homocysteine and arterial occlusive disease: A Concise Review, Cardiologia, 44(4), pp341–345, 1999.

12. Walker, R., If I eat another carrot I'll go crazy!, Kingsclear Books, Crows Nest, Sydney, 1996.

13. Walker, R., What's Cookin' Doc?, Kingsclear Books, Crows Nest, Sydney, 1998.

14. Cranton, E. M., A Textbook on EDTA Chelation Therapy, Human Sciences Press, INC, New York, 1989.

CHAPTER 5.

1. Goldman, R., Brain Fitness: Anti-Ageing Strategies for achieving Super Mind Power, Doubleday, New York, 1999.

2. Crook, T. H. and Adderly, B., The Memory Cure, Pocket Books, New York, 1998.

3. Hoffer, A., Alzheimer's: An Anecdote, Townsend Letter, 179, pp107–109, June 1998.

4. Progress report on Alzheimer's Disease, US Department of Health and Human Services, National Institute of Health, Silver Spring Md.

5. Vitamin E may help ageing memory, Journal of the American Geriatrics Society, 46, pp1407–1410, November 1998.

6. Kawas, C.S. et al., A prospective study of oestrogen replacement therapy and the risk of developing Alzheimer's Disease, The Baltimore Longitudinal Study of Ageing, Neurology, 48 (6), pp1517–1521, 1997.

7. O'Brien, J. T. and Levy, R., Age-Associated Memory Impairment: Too broad an entity to justify drug treatment Yet, British Medical Journal, 304 (6818), pp5-6, 1992.

Additional Resources
1. Crook, T. H., Treatment of Age-Related Cognitive Decline: Effects of Phosphatidylserine, Anti-Ageing Medical Therapeutics, Volume 2, pp20–29, 1998.
2. Kidd, P. M., Phosphatidylserine: The nutrient building block that accelerated all brain functions and counters Alzheimer's, A Keats Good Health Guide, 1998.
3. Burke, E. R., Phosphatidylserine: Promise for athletic performance, A Keats Good Health Guide, 1998.

CHAPTER 6.

1. American Institute for Cancer Research, Food, Nutrition & Cancer: A Global Perspective, Banta Book Group, Menasha, WI, 1997.
2. Dean, W., Can DHEA Prevent BPH and prostate cancer?, Townsend Letter, 180, p33, July 1998.
3. Clorfene-Casten, L., Breast cancer: Poisons, profits and prevention, Townsend Letter, 178, pp24–31, May 1998.
4. Pelton, R., How to prevent breast cancer, The Science of Anti-Ageing Medicine, pp205–209, 1996.
5. Mediavilla, M.D., Melatonin Increases P53, Pub Med Life Sci, 65(47), pp415–420, 1999.
6. Zeligs, M.A., Safer estrogen with phytonutrition, Townsend Letter, 189, pp83–88, April 1999.
7. Bradlow, H.I. et al., Effects of indol-3-carbinol on estradiol metabolism and spontaneous mammary tumors in mice, Carcinogenesis, 12, pp1571–1574.

Additional Resources
1. Stephens, F.O., Phyto-oestrogens and prostate cancer: Possible preventive role, MJA, 167 (3), pp138–139, August 1997.
2. Howes, L., Isoflavone Phyto-Oestrogens, Medical Observer Update, March 1999.
3. Adlercreutz, H., Phyto-Oestrogens: Epidemiology and a possible role in cancer prevention, Environmental Health Perspectives, 103 (7), pp103–112, 1995.
4. Morton, M.S. et al., The preventive role of diet in prostatic disease, British Journal of Urology, 77, pp481–493, 1996.

5. Novogen, NV-06 A new drug with potent activity against both prostatic activity and prostatic enlargement, June 1999.
6. Doneo-Pellegrini, H. et al., Foods, Nutrients and prostate cancer: a case control study in Uruguay, Br J Cancer, 80 (3-4), pp591–597, 1999.
7. Liang, J.Y. et al., Inhibitory effect of zinc on human prostatic cancer cell growth, Prostate, 40 (3), pp200–207, 1999.
8. Rao, K.V. et al., Chemoprevention of rat prostate carcinogenesis by early and delayed administration of DHEA, Cancer Res, 59 (13), pp3084–3089, 1999.
9. Stephens, F.O., The rising incidence of breast cancer in women and prostate cancer in men. Dietary Influences: A possible preventive role for nature's sex hormone modifiers—The Phyto-Oestrogens, Oncol Rep, 6 (4), pp865–870, 1999.
10. Levy, J. and Regtop, H., Preventative cancer review, Bullivants Lecture Series, 1997.
11. Buist, R., Cancer: Prevention and treatment, Pharma Foods Lecture Series, 1999.

CHAPTER 7.

1.&4.&9.&13. Taylor, M., Alternatives to conventional hormone replacement therapy, Comp Ther, 23 (8), pp514–532, 1997.
2. Eden, J. A., Women's hormone problems, 1995.
3.&6 Wright, J.V. and, J., Natural Hormone Replacement, Smart Publications, Petaluma, CA, 1997.
5.&7.&10. Eden, J.A., Managing menopause: HRT or herbal? Modern Medicine, 42 (8), pp32–39, 1999.
8. Schneider, D.L. et al., Timing of postmenopausal estrogen for optimal bone mineral density, the Rancho Bernado Study, JAMA, 277, pp543–547, 1997.
11. Padwick, M.L. et al., Oestriol with Oestradiol versus oestrdiol alone: A comparison of endometrial, symptomatic and psychological features, Br J. Obstet Gynaecol, 93, p606, 1986.
14.&15. Wright, J.V. and Lenard, L., Maximise your vitality and potency, Smart Publications, Petaluma, CA, 1999.

Additional Resources

1. Beckham, H., Natural Therapies for Menopause and osteoporosis, 1997.
2. Carruthers, M., Maximising Manhood: Beating the Male Menopause, Harper Collins, London, 1996.
3. Prior, J.C., Perimenopause: The complex endocrinology of the menopausal transition, Endocrine Reviews, 19 (4), pp397–428, 1998.
4. Clinical Synthesis Panel Issues Comprehensive Report on the Benefits and Risks of HRT, Lancet Report on the Internet, 354, pp152–155, 1999.
5. Delmas, P. Lectures presented at Menopause Seminar, Royal Hospital for Women, 1999.
6. Wren, B., Lectures presented at Menopause Seminar, Royal Hospital for Women. 1999.
7. Hormones and Natural Therapies Symposium, The Sydney Menopause Centre, 1998.
8. Lee, J.R., What Your Doctor May Not Tell You About Menopause, Warner Books, New York, 1996.
9. Tunstall-Pedoe, H., Myth and paradox of coronary risk and the menopause, Lancet, 351, pp1425–1427, 1998.
10. Wilson, P.W.F. et al., Postmenopausal oestrogen use and cigarette smoking and cardiovascular morbidity in women over 50, The Framingham study. NEJM, 313 (17), pp1038–1043, 1985.
11. Purdie, D.W., The spectrum of Oestrogen activity, Centre for Metabolic Diseases, Hull Royal Infirmary, 1999.
12. Lieberman, S., Phytohormones in women's health: The prevention of breast cancer and the treatment of menopause, Presentation at the annual International Conference of the American Academy of Anti-ageing Medicine, Chicago, June 1999.
13. Lichten, E., Women's Anti-Ageing Medicines: Oestrogen and beyond, Presentation at the above conference.
14. Schippen, E., The Testosterone Syndrome: Male Testosterone Replacement Therapies, Presentation at the above conference.

CHAPTER 8.

1. & 8. Colgan, M., Hormonal Health, Apple Publishing, Vancouver, 1996.
2. & 5 Goldman, R., Brain Fitness, Doubleday, New York, 1999.
3., 4. & 11. Wright, J.V. and Lenard, L., Maximise your vitality and potency, Smart Publications, Petaluma, CA, 1999.
6. & 7. Hutchinson, K.A., Androgens and sexuality, The American Journal of Medicine, 98 (1S), pp1A–1159, 1995.
9. Mediherb monitor, December 1994.
10. O'Neil, J., Sex drive tied to critical substance, Journal of Longevity, 4 (9), pp19–21, 1998.
12. Lamm, S., Younger At Last, Pocket Books, New York, 1997.

Additional Resources

1. Jensen, B., Love, Sex and Nutrition, Avery Publishing Group, New York, 1998.
2. Moir, A. and Jessel, D., Brainsex, Mandarin, London, 1998.
3. Morgenthaler, J. and Joy, D., Better sex through chemistry, Smart Publications, Petaluma, CA, 1994.
4. Murray, M., Male Sexual Vitality, Prima Publishing, Rocklin, CA, 1994.
5. Walker, M., Sexual Nutrition, Avery Publishing Group, New York, 1994.
6. Hoffman, D.L., Herbal Materia Medica.
7. Morgan, M. and Bone, K., Tribulus Terrestris, Mediherb Materia Medica, 1999.
8. Sapolsky, R.M., Why zebras don't get ulcers, W.H. Freeman and Co, New York, 1998.
9. Duckett, M.J., The Scientific Sexual Revolution: Sexual dysfunction and the new 'viagra like' drugs, Presentation at the annual International Conference of the American Academy of Anti-Ageing Medicine, Chicago, June 1999.

CHAPTER 9.

1. Anhalt, H., Childhood Obesity—The epidemic of the 21st Century and how it relates to premature ageing, Anti-ageing Medical Therapeutics, 2, pp60–70, 1998.

Additional Resources
2. Ahmed, A.J., Fat cells, weight regulation and obesity, Anti-ageing Medical Therapeutics, 1, pp214–218, 1998.

CHAPTER 10.

1. Evans, W. and Rosenberg, M.D., Biomarkers: The 10 keys to prolong vitality, Simon & Schuster, New York, 1991.
2. Yanick, P., Nutritional modulation of mitochondrial energetics via biological terrain assessment, Anti-Ageing Medical Therapeutics, 2, pp155–174, 1998.

Compounding pharmacy that provides natural HRT creams:
Roper and Parry's Pharmacy
89–93 Keen Street, Lismore, 2480.
Ph: (02) 6621 4000.

Laboratory that provides specialised tests for digestive
and liver function:
Analytical Reference Laboratories
5 Leveson Street,
North Melbourne, 3051.
Ph: (03) 93283586.

Vitamin company that manufactures the products
mentioned in chapters six and eight:
By Nature
6/21 Wanneroo Rd,
Joondana, Western Australia, 6060.
Ph: (08) 94505856.

Index